AGING WELL

The Longevity Blueprint

Mark Rasanoe

ISBN-13: 979-8-8672-1628-3

To all those who dare to embrace the journey of aging with courage and curiosity, this book is dedicated. May you find in these pages the knowledge and inspiration to lead lives that grow richer with every passing year. Your resilience, wisdom, and the beauty you bring to the world is a testament to the art of aging well. Thank you for being our guiding stars on this path.

CONTENTS

INTRODUCTION

In a world where the concept of time seems to race ever faster, where the pursuit of youth and vitality often dominates our thoughts and actions, the quest for a long and fulfilling life has never been more relevant. "Aging Well: The Longevity Blueprint" is not just another book on growing older; it is a roadmap to navigating the intricate and often mysterious journey of aging with grace, vitality, and wisdom.

In these pages, we embark on a scientific and practical exploration of the art of aging well, driven by the latest research and a commitment to honesty and directness. This book does not sugarcoat the challenges that come with growing older, nor does it dwell on empty promises or unfounded myths. Instead, it equips you with the knowledge and strategies you need to forge your own path towards a long and healthy life.

Drawing upon a vast tapestry of knowledge, from the intricacies of cellular aging to the profound impact of our daily choices, "Aging Well: The Longevity Blueprint" unveils the secrets to embracing the golden years with vigor and vitality. We will delve into the core principles of nutrition, exercise, mental health, sleep, and disease prevention, offering you a comprehensive guide to understanding and optimizing these crucial facets of your life.

But aging is not solely about numbers or measurements; it's also a deeply personal journey, unique to each of us. This book explores the emotional and psychological dimensions of growing older, focusing on the importance of maintaining cognitive function, managing stress, and nurturing your emotional well-being. It acknowledges the significance of social connections and offers strategies to keep your mind sharp and your spirits high.

In the pursuit of a long and meaningful life, sleep is often overlooked, yet it plays a vital role in our well-being. We'll provide practical solutions for addressing common sleep issues, allowing you to enhance the quality of your rest and energize your days.

Preventing age-related diseases and managing chronic conditions are challenges that confront many of us as we age. This book offers guidance and insights on how to face these hurdles with knowledge and resilience, empowering you to take control of your health and quality of life.

The journey through these pages is not merely about extending our existence but also about embracing the wisdom, resilience, and beauty that come with age. We explore the cutting-edge developments in anti-aging research, longevity technologies, and therapies, giving you a glimpse into the exciting possibilities that the future holds.

As we guide you through this comprehensive blueprint, we offer actionable advice, clear pathways, and the tools you need to make informed decisions about your own journey of aging. "Aging Well: The Longevity Blueprint" is your companion, your source of wisdom, and your partner in the pursuit of a long, healthy, and fulfilling life. It is an unapologetic and straightforward resource for those who seek to age well, welcoming the beauty and wisdom of each passing year.

1. UNDERSTANDING AGING

1.1 THE SCIENCE OF AGING

Aging is a natural process that every living organism experiences. It is a complex phenomenon that involves a multitude of biological, physiological, and psychological changes over time. In recent years, there has been a growing interest in understanding the science behind aging and how we can age well.

1.1.1 The Basics of Aging

To understand the science of aging, it is important to first grasp the basic concepts. At its core, aging is the result of a gradual decline in the body's ability to repair and regenerate cells and tissues. This decline is influenced by a variety of factors, including genetics, lifestyle choices, and environmental factors.

1.1.2 Cellular Aging

At the cellular level, aging is characterized by a progressive loss of function and integrity. One of the key theories of cellular aging is the telomere theory, which suggests that the shortening of telomeres (the protective caps at the ends of chromosomes) plays a significant role in the aging process. As telomeres shorten, cells become less able to divide and replicate, leading to cellular senescence.

Another important aspect of cellular aging is the accumulation of damage to DNA, proteins, and other cellular components. This damage can result from a variety of factors, including oxidative stress, inflammation, and exposure to toxins. Over time, the accumulation of cellular damage can impair cellular function and contribute to the aging process.

1.1.3 The Role of Genetics

While genetics play a role in the aging process, it is important to note that they are not the sole determinant of how we age. While some individuals may be genetically predisposed to age-related diseases or conditions, lifestyle choices and environmental factors can greatly influence the rate at which these conditions manifest.

Recent research has also highlighted the role of epigenetics in aging. Epigenetics refers to changes in gene expression that are not caused by alterations in the DNA sequence itself. These changes can be influenced by a variety of factors, including diet, exercise, stress, and environmental exposures. By understanding the role of epigenetics, we can better appreciate the impact of lifestyle choices on the aging process.

1.1.4 Theories of Aging

Scientists have proposed several theories to explain the underlying mechanisms of aging. One prominent theory is the mitochondrial theory of aging, which suggests that age-related decline is driven by the accumulation of damage to mitochondria, the energy-producing organelles within cells. As mitochondrial function declines, cells become less efficient at producing energy, leading to a decline in overall cellular function.

Another theory is the free radical theory of aging, which proposes that the accumulation of reactive oxygen species (ROS) and oxidative damage contributes to the aging process. ROS are highly reactive molecules that can damage cellular components, including DNA, proteins, and lipids. Over time, the accumulation of oxidative damage can impair cellular function and contribute to the aging process.

1.1.5 Longevity Genes and Aging

While genetics alone cannot determine how we age, certain genes have been identified that are associated with longevity. These genes, often referred to as "longevity genes," are believed to play a role in protecting against age-related diseases and promoting healthy aging.

One example of a longevity gene is the FOXO3 gene, which has been associated with a longer lifespan and a reduced risk of age-related diseases such as cardiovascular disease and cancer. Other longevity genes, such as SIRT1 and mTOR, have also been implicated in the aging process and are the subject of ongoing research.

1.1.6 The Impact of Lifestyle Choices

While genetics and cellular processes play a role in aging, lifestyle choices can greatly influence the rate at which we age. Research has consistently shown that adopting healthy habits, such as eating a nutritious diet, engaging in regular physical activity, managing stress, and getting adequate sleep, can have a profound impact on the aging process.

A healthy lifestyle can help to mitigate the effects of cellular aging by reducing oxidative stress, inflammation, and cellular damage. It can also promote the maintenance of healthy cellular function and support the body's natural repair and regeneration processes.

1.1.7 The Future of Aging Research

As our understanding of the science of aging continues to evolve, so too does the potential for interventions that can slow down or even reverse the aging process. Scientists are exploring a variety of approaches, including the use of senolytics to remove senescent cells, the development of anti-aging drugs, and the exploration of regenerative medicine techniques.

While these advancements hold promise, it is important to approach them with caution and skepticism. Aging is a complex process, and there is still much to learn about the underlying mechanisms and potential interventions. In the meantime, adopting a healthy lifestyle remains the most effective strategy for aging well.

In the following chapters, we will delve deeper into the factors that affect aging, including nutrition, exercise, mental health, sleep, and the prevention of age-related diseases. By understanding the science of aging and implementing evidence-based strategies, we can optimize our health and well-being as we age.

1.2 FACTORS AFFECTING AGING

Aging is a complex process influenced by a variety of factors. While some aspects of aging are inevitable and determined by our genetic makeup, there are several factors that can significantly impact how we age. Understanding these factors is crucial for developing a comprehensive plan to age well and maintain optimal health and vitality.

1.2.1 Genetic Factors

Our genes play a significant role in determining how we age. Some individuals may be genetically predisposed to age-related diseases or conditions, while others may have genes that promote longevity and healthy aging. Genetic factors can influence various aspects of aging, including the rate at which our cells age, the efficiency of our body's repair mechanisms, and our susceptibility to age-related diseases.

While we cannot change our genetic makeup, understanding our genetic predispositions can help us make informed decisions about our lifestyle choices and healthcare. Genetic testing and counseling can provide valuable insights into our individual genetic risks and guide us in making proactive choices to mitigate those risks.

1.2.2 Lifestyle Factors

Lifestyle factors have a profound impact on how we age. The choices we make regarding our diet, physical activity, sleep patterns, stress management, and social connections can significantly influence our overall health and well-being as we age.

Diet: A nutritious and balanced diet is essential for healthy aging. Consuming a variety of fruits, vegetables, whole grains, lean proteins, and healthy fats provides the necessary nutrients to support optimal bodily functions and combat age-related diseases. On the other hand, a diet high in processed foods, sugar, and unhealthy fats can accelerate the aging process and increase the risk of chronic diseases.

Physical Activity: Regular exercise is crucial for maintaining physical and mental health as we age. Engaging in aerobic exercises, strength training, and flexibility exercises can improve cardiovascular health, muscle strength, bone density, and cognitive function. Exercise also helps manage weight, reduce the risk of chronic diseases, and enhance overall well-being.

Sleep: Quality sleep is essential for cellular repair, cognitive function, and emotional well-being. Poor sleep patterns and sleep disorders can accelerate the aging process and increase the risk of age-related diseases. Establishing a healthy sleep routine and addressing any sleep issues can significantly improve the quality of our sleep and promote healthy aging.

Stress Management: Chronic stress can have detrimental effects on our physical and mental health. High levels of stress hormones can accelerate the aging process and increase the risk of age-related diseases. Adopting stress management techniques such as meditation, deep breathing exercises, and engaging in activities that promote relaxation can help mitigate the negative effects of stress and promote healthy aging.

Social Connections: Maintaining strong social connections and engaging in meaningful relationships is vital for healthy aging. Social isolation and loneliness can have detrimental effects on our mental and physical health, increasing the risk of depression, cognitive decline, and chronic diseases. Building and nurturing social connections can provide emotional support, reduce stress, and enhance overall well-being.

1.2.3 Environmental Factors

Environmental factors can also impact how we age. Our exposure to pollutants, toxins, and harmful substances in our environment can accelerate the aging process and increase the risk of age-related diseases. Additionally, factors such as air quality, access to healthcare, and socioeconomic status can influence our overall health and well-being as we age.

Pollution: Exposure to air pollution, water contamination, and other environmental toxins can have detrimental effects on our health and accelerate the aging process. Minimizing exposure to pollutants and adopting measures to improve air and water quality can help mitigate these risks.

Access to Healthcare: Access to quality healthcare plays a crucial role in healthy aging. Regular check-ups, preventive screenings, and timely medical interventions can help detect and manage age-related diseases effectively. Ensuring access to healthcare services and staying proactive in managing our health can significantly impact how we age.

Socioeconomic Factors: Socioeconomic factors, such as income, education, and social support, can influence our ability to adopt healthy lifestyle choices and access healthcare services. Individuals with higher socioeconomic status often have better access to resources and opportunities that promote healthy aging.

1.2.4 Psychological Factors

Psychological factors, such as our mindset, attitude, and resilience, can also impact how we age. Research suggests that individuals with a positive outlook on aging tend to have better physical and mental health outcomes compared to those with negative perceptions of aging.

Embracing a positive mindset, cultivating resilience, and maintaining a sense of purpose and meaning in life can contribute to healthy aging.

Aging is a multifaceted process influenced by a combination of genetic, lifestyle, environmental, and psychological factors. While we cannot control all aspects of aging, understanding these factors empowers us to make informed choices that can positively impact our health and well-being as we age. By adopting a comprehensive approach that addresses these factors, we can create a blueprint for aging well and enjoying a long and fulfilling life.

1.3 COMMON AGING MYTHS

As we age, there are many myths and misconceptions that surround the process of getting older. These myths can often lead to misunderstandings and unnecessary fears about aging. In this section, we will debunk some of the most common aging myths and provide you with accurate information to help you better understand the aging process.

1.3.1 Myth: Aging is solely determined by genetics

One of the most prevalent myths about aging is

that it is solely determined by our genetics. While genetics do play a role in how we age, they are not the sole determining factor. Research has shown that lifestyle choices, such as diet, exercise, and stress management, can have a significant impact on the aging process. By adopting healthy habits, we can positively influence our overall health and well-being as we age.

1.3.2 Myth: Aging means inevitable decline

Another common myth is that aging inevitably leads to a decline in physical and mental abilities. While it is true that certain changes occur as we age, such as a decrease in muscle mass and cognitive function, it does not mean that we are destined to experience a decline in overall health. With proper care and attention to our physical and mental well-being, we can maintain and even improve our quality of life as we age.

1.3.3 Myth: Older adults should avoid exercise

Contrary to popular belief, exercise is not only safe but highly beneficial for older adults. Regular physical activity can help maintain muscle strength, improve balance and coordination, and reduce the risk of chronic diseases such as heart disease and diabetes. It is important to engage in a variety of exercises that focus on cardiovascular fitness, strength training, and flexibility to promote overall health and well-being.

1.3.4 Myth: Aging means becoming forgetful

While it is true that some degree of memory decline can occur with age, it is not an inevitable part of the aging process. Many older adults maintain excellent cognitive function well into their later years. Engaging in mentally stimulating activities, such as puzzles, reading, and learning new skills, can help keep the mind sharp and reduce the risk of cognitive decline.

1.3.5 Myth: Older adults should eat less

Another common myth is that older adults should eat less as they age. While it is true that our metabolism slows down as we get older, it is important to maintain a balanced and nutritious diet to support overall health. Older adults should focus on consuming nutrient-dense foods that provide essential vitamins, minerals, and antioxidants. Adequate protein intake is also crucial for maintaining muscle mass and strength.

1.3.6 Myth: Aging means being lonely and isolated

Contrary to popular belief, aging does not automatically mean being lonely and isolated. While it is true that social connections may change as we age, it is important to prioritize maintaining and nurturing relationships. Engaging in social activities, joining clubs or organizations, and staying connected with family and friends can help combat feelings of loneliness and promote overall well-being.

1.3.7 Myth: Aging means losing interest in sex

Another common myth is that older adults lose interest in sex. While it is true that sexual desire and function may change with age, many older adults continue to enjoy a fulfilling and satisfying sex life. Open communication with a partner, maintaining overall health, and addressing any physical or emotional concerns can help ensure a healthy and enjoyable sexual relationship as we age.

1.3.8 Myth: Aging means being dependent on others

A common misconception is that aging automatically means being dependent on others for daily activities. While some individuals may require assistance as they age, many older adults maintain their independence and lead active and fulfilling lives. By adopting healthy lifestyle habits, managing chronic conditions, and seeking appropriate support when needed, older adults can maintain their independence and autonomy.

1.3.9 Myth: Aging means losing purpose and meaning

Contrary to popular belief, aging does not mean losing purpose and meaning in life. Many older adults find new passions, hobbies, and interests as they age, and continue to contribute to their communities and society. It is important to embrace the opportunities that come with aging and find ways to stay engaged and fulfilled, whether through volunteering, pursuing creative endeavors, or spending time with loved ones.

1.3.10 Myth: Aging means being unhappy

Lastly, a common myth is that aging means being unhappy. While it is true that older adults may face unique challenges and experiences, research has shown that overall life satisfaction tends to increase with age. Older adults often have a greater sense of wisdom, resilience, and gratitude, which can contribute to a more positive outlook on life. By focusing on maintaining physical and mental well-being, older adults can continue to experience happiness and fulfillment as they age.

In conclusion, it is important to separate fact from fiction when it comes to aging. By debunking these common aging myths, we can better understand the aging process and take proactive steps to age well. Aging is a natural part of life, and with the right knowledge and strategies, we can embrace the journey and enjoy a long and healthy life.

1.4 THE AGING PROCESS EXPLAINED

Aging is a natural and inevitable process that every living organism experiences. It is a complex phenomenon that involves a gradual decline in the body's ability to function and repair itself. While aging is a universal process, the rate at which it occurs can vary from person to person. Understanding the aging process is crucial for developing strategies to promote healthy aging and enhance longevity.

1.4.1 Cellular Aging

At the core of the aging process is cellular aging. Our bodies are made up of trillions of cells, each with a specific function. Over time, these cells undergo changes that affect their structure and function. One of the key factors contributing to cellular aging is the shortening of telomeres, which are protective caps at the ends of our chromosomes. Telomeres naturally shorten with each cell division, and when they become too short, cells can no longer divide and function properly.

Another important aspect of cellular aging is the

accumulation of damage to cellular components, such as DNA, proteins, and lipids. This damage can be caused by various factors, including oxidative stress, inflammation, and exposure to environmental toxins. As cells accumulate damage, their ability to function efficiently decreases, leading to the overall decline in organ and tissue function that is characteristic of aging.

1.4.2 Hormonal Changes

Hormonal changes also play a significant role in the aging process. As we age, the production and regulation of hormones in our bodies undergo changes. For example, the production of growth hormone, which is essential for tissue repair and regeneration, decreases with age. This decline in growth hormone production can contribute to the loss of muscle mass and strength commonly observed in older adults.

Similarly, the production of sex hormones, such as estrogen and testosterone, declines with age. These hormones play crucial roles in maintaining bone density, muscle mass, and sexual function. The decline in sex hormone production can lead to conditions such as osteoporosis and loss of libido.

1.4.3 Genetic Factors

Genetics also influence the aging process. Certain

genetic variations can predispose individuals to age-related diseases and affect their overall rate of aging. For example, variations in genes involved in DNA repair mechanisms can impact the body's ability to repair DNA damage, leading to accelerated aging.

Additionally, genetic factors can influence the production and activity of antioxidant enzymes, which help protect cells from oxidative damage. Variations in these genes can affect an individual's susceptibility to oxidative stress and contribute to the aging process.

1.4.4 Lifestyle Factors

While genetics and cellular changes play a significant role in aging, lifestyle factors also have a profound impact on the aging process. Unhealthy lifestyle habits, such as poor nutrition, lack of exercise, chronic stress, and inadequate sleep, can accelerate the aging process and increase the risk of age-related diseases.

On the other hand, adopting a healthy lifestyle can slow down the aging process and promote longevity. A balanced diet rich in nutrients, regular physical activity, stress management techniques, and sufficient sleep can all contribute to healthy aging. These lifestyle factors can help reduce oxidative stress, inflammation, and cellular damage, thereby slowing down the aging process at a cellular level.

1.4.5 The Role of Inflammation

Inflammation is a natural immune response that helps the body fight off infections and repair damaged tissues. However, chronic inflammation, which persists over an extended period, can contribute to the aging process. Chronic inflammation can damage cells and tissues, leading to the development of age-related diseases such as cardiovascular disease, diabetes, and neurodegenerative disorders.

Various factors, including poor diet, sedentary lifestyle, obesity, and chronic stress, can contribute to chronic inflammation. By adopting a healthy lifestyle and implementing strategies to reduce inflammation, such as consuming anti-inflammatory foods and practicing stress management techniques, individuals can mitigate the negative effects of chronic inflammation and promote healthy aging.

1.4.6 The Role of Oxidative Stress

Oxidative stress is another key factor in the aging process. It occurs when there is an imbalance between the production of reactive oxygen species (ROS) and the body's antioxidant defenses. ROS are highly reactive molecules that can damage cells and contribute to the aging process.

Various factors, including exposure to environmental toxins, poor diet, smoking, and excessive alcohol consumption, can increase the production of ROS and overwhelm the body's antioxidant defenses. This can lead to oxidative damage to cells and tissues, accelerating the aging process.

To combat oxidative stress and promote healthy aging, it is important to consume a diet rich in antioxidants, such as fruits, vegetables, and whole grains. Antioxidants help neutralize ROS and protect cells from oxidative damage.

1.4.7 The Importance of Genetic and Environmental Interactions

It is important to note that the aging process is not solely determined by genetics or lifestyle factors but is a complex interplay between the two. While genetics can influence an individual's susceptibility to age-related diseases and the rate of aging, lifestyle factors can modulate the expression of genes and influence how they impact the aging process.

Furthermore, environmental factors, such as exposure to pollutants and toxins, can interact with genetic factors and accelerate the aging process. Understanding these interactions is crucial for developing personalized strategies to promote healthy aging and enhance longevity.

The aging process is a multifaceted phenomenon influenced by cellular changes, hormonal fluctuations, genetic factors, and lifestyle choices. By understanding the underlying mechanisms of aging, individuals can make informed decisions and implement strategies to promote healthy aging and enhance longevity.

2. NUTRITION AND AGING

2.1 THE ROLE OF NUTRITION IN LONGEVITY

Nutrition plays a crucial role in our overall health and well-being, and it becomes even more important as we age. The food we consume provides the necessary nutrients for our bodies to function optimally and maintain a strong immune system. In this section, we will explore the role of nutrition in longevity and how making informed dietary choices can positively impact our health as we age.

2.1.1 The Link Between Nutrition and Longevity

Research has consistently shown that a well-balanced diet can significantly contribute to a longer and healthier life. The nutrients we obtain from food are essential for maintaining the proper functioning of our organs, tissues, and cells. They provide the building blocks for our bodies to repair and regenerate, which becomes increasingly important as we age.

A diet rich in fruits, vegetables, whole grains, lean proteins, and healthy fats can help reduce the risk of chronic diseases such as heart disease, diabetes, and certain types of cancer. These diseases are often associated with aging, and by adopting a nutritious diet, we can potentially delay their onset and improve our overall quality of life.

2.1.2 Key Nutrients for Healthy Aging

While a balanced diet is important, certain nutrients have been specifically linked to healthy aging. Let's explore some of these key nutrients and their benefits:

Omega-3 Fatty Acids

Omega-3 fatty acids, found in fatty fish like salmon and sardines, as well as walnuts and flaxseeds, have been shown to have numerous health benefits. They can help reduce inflammation, lower the risk of heart disease, and support brain health. Including omega-3 fatty acids in our diet can contribute to maintaining cognitive function and reducing the risk of age-related cognitive decline.

Antioxidants

Antioxidants are compounds that help protect our cells from damage caused by free radicals, which are unstable molecules that can contribute to aging and disease. Foods rich in antioxidants, such as berries, dark chocolate, and leafy greens, can help reduce oxidative stress and inflammation in the body. By including these foods in our diet, we can support our immune system and reduce the risk of chronic diseases.

Fiber

Fiber is essential for maintaining a healthy digestive system and preventing constipation, a common issue among older adults. It can also help regulate blood sugar levels and lower cholesterol, reducing the risk of heart disease. Including fiber-rich foods like whole grains, legumes, fruits, and vegetables in our diet can promote healthy digestion and support overall well-being.

Calcium and Vitamin D

As we age, maintaining strong bones becomes increasingly important to prevent conditions like osteoporosis. Calcium and vitamin D are crucial for bone health, as calcium provides the building blocks for bones, and vitamin D helps with calcium absorption. Dairy products, leafy greens, and fortified foods are excellent sources of calcium, while sunlight exposure and fatty fish can provide us with vitamin D.

2.1.3 Eating Well for Longevity

Adopting a healthy eating pattern is essential for promoting longevity and overall well-being. Here are some practical tips for eating well as we age:

Focus on Whole Foods

Prioritize whole, unprocessed foods in your diet. These include fruits, vegetables, whole grains, lean proteins, and healthy fats. These foods are rich in essential nutrients and provide the necessary fuel for our bodies to function optimally.

Practice Portion Control

As we age, our metabolism tends to slow down, and our calorie needs may decrease. It's important to be mindful of portion sizes to maintain a healthy weight. Use smaller plates and bowls, and listen to your body's hunger and fullness cues.

Stay Hydrated

Dehydration can be a common issue among older adults, as our sense of thirst may diminish with age. Make sure to drink an adequate amount of water throughout the day to stay hydrated. Limit the consumption of sugary beverages and alcohol, as they can contribute to dehydration.

Limit Processed Foods and Added Sugars

Processed foods often contain high levels of unhealthy fats, sodium, and added sugars. These can contribute to inflammation, weight gain, and an increased risk of chronic diseases. Opt for whole, unprocessed foods whenever possible and limit your intake of sugary snacks and beverages.

Seek Professional Guidance

If you have specific dietary concerns or health conditions, it's advisable to consult with a registered dietitian or healthcare professional. They can provide personalized recommendations based on your individual needs and help you create a nutrition plan that supports healthy aging.

2.1.4 Meal Planning for Aging Well

Meal planning can be a helpful strategy for ensuring a nutritious and balanced diet. Here are some tips for effective meal planning:

Plan Ahead

Take some time each week to plan your meals and create a shopping list. This will help you stay organized and ensure that you have all the necessary ingredients on hand.

Include a Variety of Foods

Aim to include a variety of foods from different food groups in your meals. This will ensure that you obtain a wide range of nutrients and prevent dietary monotony.

Cook in Batches

Consider cooking larger portions and storing leftovers for future meals. This can save time and effort, especially on busy days when you may not have the energy to cook a full meal.

Experiment with New Recipes

Try incorporating new recipes and flavors into your meal plan. This can make healthy eating more enjoyable and prevent boredom with your diet.

Be Mindful of Special Dietary Needs

If you have specific dietary restrictions or allergies, make sure to plan meals that accommodate these needs. There are plenty of resources available for finding delicious recipes that cater to various dietary preferences.

By understanding the role of nutrition in longevity and making conscious choices about what we eat, we can support our overall health and well-being as we age. A nutritious diet, combined with other healthy lifestyle habits, can contribute to a longer, healthier, and more fulfilling life.

2.2 COMMON EXECUTION CHALLENGES

Eating well is a crucial component of aging well. The food we consume plays a significant role in our overall health and can greatly impact our longevity. In this section, we will explore the importance of nutrition in promoting healthy aging and provide practical tips for incorporating a nutritious diet into your daily life.

2.3.1 The Power of a Balanced Diet

A balanced diet is essential for maintaining optimal health as we age. It provides the necessary nutrients, vitamins, and minerals that our bodies need to function properly. A well-rounded diet consists of a variety of foods from different food groups, including fruits, vegetables, whole grains, lean proteins, and healthy fats.

Fruits and vegetables are rich in antioxidants, which help protect our cells from damage caused by free radicals. They also provide essential vitamins and minerals that support various bodily functions. Aim to include a colorful array of fruits and vegetables in your meals to ensure you are getting a wide range of nutrients.

Whole grains, such as brown rice, quinoa, and whole wheat bread, are excellent sources of fiber, which aids in digestion and helps regulate blood sugar levels. Fiber also promotes a feeling of fullness, which can prevent overeating and aid in weight management.

Lean proteins, such as fish, poultry, beans, and tofu, are important for maintaining muscle mass and supporting overall body function. They are also rich in essential amino acids, which are the building blocks of proteins and play a vital role in repairing and maintaining tissues.

Healthy fats, such as those found in avocados, nuts, and olive oil, are beneficial for heart health and can help reduce the risk of chronic diseases. These fats also aid in the absorption of fat-soluble vitamins, such as vitamins A, D, E, and K.

2.3.2 The Mediterranean Diet: A Model for Longevity

One dietary pattern that has been extensively studied for its health benefits is the Mediterranean diet. This eating plan is inspired by the traditional dietary patterns of countries bordering the Mediterranean Sea, such as Greece and Italy.

The Mediterranean diet emphasizes the consumption of fruits, vegetables, whole grains, legumes, nuts, seeds, and olive oil. It also includes moderate amounts of fish, poultry, and dairy products, while limiting red meat and processed foods.

Numerous studies have shown that following a Mediterranean diet can reduce the risk of heart disease, stroke, and certain types of cancer. It is also associated with a lower incidence of age-related cognitive decline and a longer lifespan.

To adopt a Mediterranean-style eating pattern, incorporate the following principles into your diet:

Eat plenty of fruits and vegetables: Aim for at least five servings of fruits and vegetables per day. Include a variety of colors to ensure a wide range of nutrients.
Choose whole grains: Opt for whole grain bread, pasta, and rice instead of refined grains. These provide more fiber and nutrients.
Include healthy fats: Use olive oil as your primary cooking oil and incorporate nuts, seeds, and avocados into your meals.
Consume lean proteins: Include fish, poultry, beans, and legumes as your main sources of protein. Limit red meat consumption.
Moderate dairy intake: Choose low-fat dairy products, such as yogurt and cheese, in moderation.
Limit processed foods and added sugars: Minimize the consumption of processed foods, sugary beverages, and sweets.

2.3.3 Hydration and Aging

Staying hydrated is essential for overall health

and plays a vital role in healthy aging. As we age, our sense of thirst may diminish, making it easier to become dehydrated. Dehydration can lead to various health issues, including fatigue, dizziness, and impaired cognitive function.

To ensure adequate hydration, aim to drink at least eight glasses of water per day. You can also obtain hydration from other sources, such as herbal teas, infused water, and fruits with high water content, like watermelon and cucumbers.

It's important to note that individual hydration needs may vary based on factors such as activity level, climate, and overall health. If you have specific medical conditions or take medications that affect fluid balance, consult with your healthcare provider for personalized hydration recommendations.

2.3.4 Practical Tips for Healthy Eating

Incorporating healthy eating habits into your daily life doesn't have to be complicated. Here are some practical tips to help you eat well for longevity:

Plan your meals: Take the time to plan your meals for the week, including breakfast, lunch, dinner, and snacks. This will help you make healthier choices and avoid impulsive, unhealthy food choices.

Cook at home: Cooking your meals at home allows you to have control over the ingredients and portion sizes. Experiment with new recipes and try to incorporate a variety of nutritious foods into your meals.

Practice mindful eating: Slow down and savor each bite. Pay attention to your body's hunger and fullness cues. This can help prevent overeating and promote better digestion.

Include a variety of colors: Aim to have a colorful plate by including a variety of fruits and vegetables. Different colors indicate different nutrients, so the more variety, the better.

Limit processed foods: Processed foods are often high in unhealthy fats, added sugars, and sodium. Try to minimize your intake of processed snacks, fast food, and pre-packaged meals.

Practice portion control: Be mindful of portion sizes to avoid overeating. Use smaller plates and bowls to help control portion sizes visually.

Stay consistent: Consistency is key when it comes to healthy eating. Aim to make nutritious choices most of the time, but also allow yourself to enjoy occasional treats in moderation.

By following these tips and adopting a balanced, Mediterranean-inspired diet, you can nourish your body and promote healthy aging from the inside out. Remember, small changes can make a big difference in your overall health and longevity.

3. EXERCISE AND AGING

3.1 BENEFITS OF EXERCISE FOR AGING

Exercise is a crucial component of healthy aging. It offers numerous benefits that can enhance physical, mental, and emotional well-being. Regular physical activity has been shown to improve overall health, increase longevity, and reduce the risk of chronic diseases commonly associated with aging. In this section, we will explore the specific benefits of exercise for aging and why it should be an integral part of your longevity blueprint.

3.1.1 Physical Health Benefits

1. Maintaining Muscle Mass and Strength

As we age, we naturally lose muscle mass and strength, a condition known as sarcopenia. Regular exercise, particularly resistance training, can help counteract this process by stimulating muscle growth and preserving muscle mass. By maintaining strong muscles, you can improve your balance, stability, and overall physical function, reducing the risk of falls and injuries.

2. Enhancing Bone Health

Osteoporosis, a condition characterized by weak and brittle bones, is a common concern among older adults. Engaging in weight-bearing exercises, such as walking, jogging, or weightlifting, can help strengthen bones and reduce the risk of fractures. Exercise also promotes the production of osteoblasts, the cells responsible for bone formation, leading to improved bone density and overall bone health.

3. Improving Cardiovascular Fitness

Regular aerobic exercise, such as brisk walking, cycling, or swimming, can significantly improve cardiovascular fitness. It strengthens the heart muscle, lowers blood pressure, and improves blood circulation. By enhancing cardiovascular health, exercise reduces the risk of heart disease, stroke, and other cardiovascular conditions, which are more prevalent in older adults.

4. Managing Weight and Metabolism

Maintaining a healthy weight becomes increasingly challenging as we age due to changes in metabolism and hormonal fluctuations. Exercise plays a vital role in weight management by burning calories, increasing metabolism, and preserving lean muscle mass. It can also help prevent age-related weight gain and reduce the risk of obesity, which is associated with various chronic diseases.

5. Enhancing Joint Health and Flexibility

Regular exercise can help improve joint health and flexibility, reducing the risk of joint pain, stiffness, and conditions such as arthritis. Activities like yoga, tai chi, and stretching exercises can enhance joint mobility, increase range of motion, and improve overall flexibility. By keeping your joints healthy and flexible, you can maintain an active lifestyle and perform daily tasks with ease.

3.1.2 Mental and Cognitive Benefits

1. Boosting Brain Health and Cognitive Function

Exercise has been shown to have a positive impact on brain health and cognitive function. It increases blood flow to the brain, promoting the delivery of oxygen and nutrients essential for optimal brain function. Regular physical activity has been linked to improved memory, attention, and executive function. It also reduces the risk of cognitive decline and neurodegenerative diseases such as Alzheimer's and dementia.

2. Reducing the Risk of Depression and Anxiety

Mental health is equally important as physical

health for overall well-being. Exercise has been proven to be an effective natural remedy for reducing symptoms of depression and anxiety. Physical activity stimulates the release of endorphins, also known as "feel-good" hormones, which can improve mood, reduce stress, and enhance overall mental well-being. Engaging in regular exercise can provide a sense of accomplishment, boost self-esteem, and promote a positive outlook on life.

3. Improving Sleep Quality

Sleep disturbances are common among older adults, leading to fatigue, irritability, and decreased cognitive function. Regular exercise can help improve sleep quality and duration. Physical activity promotes the release of serotonin, a neurotransmitter that regulates sleep, mood, and appetite. By incorporating exercise into your daily routine, you can experience more restful and rejuvenating sleep, leading to improved overall health and well-being.

4. Enhancing Stress Management

Stress is a natural part of life, but chronic stress can have detrimental effects on physical and mental health. Exercise is a powerful stress management tool. It helps reduce the levels of stress hormones, such as cortisol, and promotes the release of endorphins, which act as natural stress relievers. Engaging in physical activity can provide a healthy outlet for stress, improve mood, and enhance resilience in the face of life's challenges.

3.1.3 Social and Emotional Benefits

1. Promoting Social Connections
Exercise can be a social activity, providing opportunities to connect with others and build meaningful relationships. Joining group exercise classes, walking clubs, or sports teams can foster a sense of community and belonging. Social interactions during exercise can combat feelings of loneliness and isolation, which are common among older adults, and contribute to overall mental well-being.

2. Enhancing Emotional Resilience
Regular exercise has been shown to enhance emotional resilience and improve overall emotional well-being. Physical activity stimulates the release of endorphins, which can elevate mood and reduce feelings of sadness or anxiety. Engaging in exercise regularly can help you better cope with life's challenges, improve self-confidence, and promote a positive outlook on aging.

Incorporating regular exercise into your daily routine is essential for healthy aging. The physical, mental, and emotional benefits of exercise are numerous and can significantly improve your overall well-being. Whether it's strength training, aerobic exercises, or activities that promote flexibility and balance, finding enjoyable ways to stay active will contribute to a long and fulfilling life.

3.2 TYPES OF EXERCISE FOR LONGEVITY

Exercise is a crucial component of healthy aging. Regular physical activity can help maintain muscle strength, improve cardiovascular health, enhance cognitive function, and boost overall well-being. However, not all exercises are created equal when it comes to promoting longevity. In this section, we will explore different types of exercises that are particularly beneficial for aging well.

3.2.1 Aerobic Exercise

Aerobic exercise, also known as cardiovascular exercise, is essential for maintaining a healthy heart and lungs. It involves activities that increase your heart rate and breathing, such as walking, jogging, swimming, cycling, or dancing. Engaging in aerobic exercise regularly can improve cardiovascular fitness, lower blood pressure, reduce the risk of heart disease, and enhance overall endurance.

One of the key benefits of aerobic exercise is its

ability to increase oxygen flow to the brain, which can enhance cognitive function and reduce the risk of age-related cognitive decline. Additionally, aerobic exercise promotes the release of endorphins, which are natural mood boosters that can help combat stress and improve mental well-being.

To incorporate aerobic exercise into your routine, aim for at least 150 minutes of moderate-intensity aerobic activity or 75 minutes of vigorous-intensity aerobic activity per week. You can start with shorter sessions and gradually increase the duration and intensity as your fitness level improves.

3.2.2 Strength Training

Strength training, also known as resistance training or weightlifting, is crucial for maintaining muscle mass and strength as we age. As we get older, we naturally lose muscle mass, which can lead to decreased mobility, increased risk of falls, and a decline in overall physical function. However, regular strength training can help counteract these effects by building and preserving muscle mass.

Strength training involves using resistance, such as dumbbells, resistance bands, or weight machines, to challenge your muscles. It can be done using various exercises that target different muscle groups, including squats, lunges, push-ups, and bicep curls. It is important to start with lighter weights and gradually increase the resistance as your muscles become stronger.

In addition to preserving muscle mass, strength training offers numerous other benefits for longevity. It can improve bone density, reduce the risk of osteoporosis, enhance joint stability, and increase metabolism. It is recommended to engage in strength training exercises at least two days a week, targeting all major muscle groups.

3.2.3 Flexibility and Balance Exercises

Flexibility and balance exercises are often overlooked but are essential for maintaining mobility and preventing falls, especially in older adults. These exercises focus on improving joint range of motion, enhancing flexibility, and enhancing balance and stability.

Yoga and Pilates are excellent examples of exercises that promote flexibility and balance. These practices involve a series of poses and movements that stretch and strengthen the muscles while also improving balance and body awareness. Tai Chi is another popular exercise that combines slow, flowing movements with deep breathing and meditation, promoting balance, flexibility, and relaxation.

Regular participation in flexibility and balance exercises can help improve posture, reduce the risk of falls, and enhance overall physical performance. It is recommended to incorporate these exercises into your routine at least two to three times a week.

3.2.4 Functional Training

Functional training focuses on exercises that mimic everyday movements and activities, improving your ability to perform daily tasks with ease. These exercises target multiple muscle groups and joints simultaneously, enhancing overall strength, flexibility, and coordination.

Examples of functional exercises include squats, lunges, step-ups, and push-ups. These exercises engage the core muscles and promote stability, which is crucial for maintaining balance and preventing falls. Functional training can also improve posture, enhance joint mobility, and increase overall functional capacity.

Incorporating functional training into your exercise routine can have a significant impact on your ability to perform daily activities independently and maintain a high quality of life as you age. Aim to include functional exercises at least two to three times a week, focusing on movements that mimic your daily activities.

3.2.5 Mind-Body Exercises

Mind-body exercises combine physical movement with mental focus and relaxation techniques, promoting both physical and mental well-being. These exercises emphasize the connection between the mind and body, helping to reduce stress, improve mood, and enhance overall mindfulness.

Yoga and Tai Chi are excellent examples of mind-body exercises. These practices involve a combination of physical postures, breathing techniques, and meditation, promoting relaxation, flexibility, and mental clarity. Mind-body exercises can also help improve sleep quality, reduce anxiety and depression, and enhance overall resilience.

Incorporating mind-body exercises into your routine can provide a holistic approach to aging well, addressing both physical and mental aspects of health. Aim to practice mind-body exercises at least two to three times a week, allowing yourself to fully immerse in the practice and reap the benefits of relaxation and mindfulness.

3.2.6 Interval Training

Interval training involves alternating between periods of high-intensity exercise and periods of rest or lower-intensity exercise. This type of exercise can be particularly beneficial for aging well as it challenges the cardiovascular system, boosts metabolism, and improves overall fitness.

High-intensity interval training (HIIT) is a popular form of interval training that involves short bursts of intense exercise followed by brief recovery periods. HIIT workouts can be adapted to various activities, such as running, cycling, or bodyweight exercises. These workouts are time-efficient and can be completed in as little as 20 minutes, making them suitable for individuals with busy schedules.

Interval training can help improve cardiovascular fitness, increase calorie burn, and enhance insulin sensitivity. It can also stimulate the production of human growth hormone (HGH), which plays a role in muscle growth and repair. However, it is important to start gradually and consult with a healthcare professional before engaging in high-intensity exercise, especially if you have any underlying health conditions.

Incorporating a variety of exercises into your routine, including aerobic exercise, strength training, flexibility and balance exercises, functional training, mind-body exercises, and interval training, can provide a well-rounded approach to promoting longevity. Remember to listen to your body, start at a comfortable level, and gradually increase the intensity and duration of your workouts. By staying active and engaging in regular exercise, you can optimize your physical and mental health as you age.

3.3 CREATING AN EXERCISE ROUTINE

Exercise is a crucial component of healthy aging. It not only helps to maintain physical fitness but also plays a significant role in preventing age-related diseases and promoting overall well-being. Creating an exercise routine that suits your needs and preferences is essential for long-term success. In this section, we will explore the key factors to consider when designing an exercise routine for aging well.

3.3.1 Setting Realistic Goals

Before starting any exercise program, it is important to set realistic goals that align with your current fitness level and overall health. Setting achievable goals will help you stay motivated and track your progress effectively. Whether your goal is to improve cardiovascular fitness, increase strength and flexibility, or simply maintain an active lifestyle, it is crucial to establish clear and attainable objectives.

3.3.2 Choosing the Right Types of Exercise

When designing an exercise routine for aging

well, it is important to incorporate a variety of exercises that target different aspects of fitness. A well-rounded routine should include cardiovascular exercises, strength training, flexibility exercises, and balance training.

Cardiovascular exercises, such as walking, swimming, or cycling, help to improve heart health, increase endurance, and boost overall fitness. Aim for at least 150 minutes of moderate-intensity aerobic activity per week, or 75 minutes of vigorous-intensity activity, spread out over several days.

Strength training exercises, such as lifting weights or using resistance bands, are crucial for maintaining muscle mass and bone density. Aim to include strength training exercises at least two days a week, targeting all major muscle groups.

Flexibility exercises, such as yoga or stretching, help to improve joint mobility and prevent injuries. Incorporate stretching exercises into your routine at least two to three times a week, focusing on all major muscle groups.

Balance training exercises, such as tai chi or standing on one leg, are important for preventing falls and maintaining stability. Include balance exercises in your routine at least two to three times a week.

3.3.3 Gradually Increasing Intensity and Duration

When starting an exercise routine, it is important to begin at a comfortable level and gradually increase the intensity and duration of your workouts. This approach allows your body to adapt and reduces the risk of injury. Start with shorter sessions and lower intensity, and gradually increase the duration and intensity as your fitness level improves.

Listen to your body and pay attention to any signs of fatigue or discomfort. If you experience pain or excessive fatigue, it is important to rest and consult with a healthcare professional if necessary. Remember, the goal is to find a balance between challenging yourself and avoiding overexertion.

3.3.4 Incorporating Variety and Enjoyment

To maintain long-term adherence to an exercise routine, it is important to incorporate variety and choose activities that you enjoy. Trying different types of exercises, such as dancing, hiking, or playing a sport, can make your routine more enjoyable and prevent boredom.

Consider joining group exercise classes or finding a workout buddy to make your exercise sessions more social and engaging. Experiment with different activities and find what works best for you. Remember, exercise should be something you look forward to, not a chore.

3.3.5 Listening to Your Body and Adapting

As we age, our bodies may have different needs and limitations. It is important to listen to your body and adapt your exercise routine accordingly. If you have any pre-existing medical conditions or physical limitations, consult with a healthcare professional or a qualified exercise specialist to ensure that your routine is safe and appropriate for your individual needs.

Be mindful of any changes in your body, such as increased joint pain or decreased flexibility, and modify your routine as necessary. It is normal for our bodies to change as we age, and adjusting our exercise routine can help us continue to stay active and healthy.

3.3.6 Staying Consistent and Overcoming Barriers

Consistency is key when it comes to reaping the benefits of exercise. Make a commitment to yourself and prioritize regular physical activity. Schedule your exercise sessions in advance and treat them as non-negotiable appointments.

Identify and overcome any barriers that may hinder your exercise routine. Lack of time, motivation, or access to facilities are common barriers that can be addressed with proper planning and creative solutions. Consider incorporating physical activity into your daily routine, such as taking the stairs instead of the elevator or going for a walk during your lunch break.

3.3.7 Seeking Professional Guidance

If you are unsure about how to design an exercise routine or have specific health concerns, it is advisable to seek professional guidance. A qualified exercise specialist, such as a certified personal trainer or a physical therapist, can provide personalized recommendations and ensure that your routine is safe and effective.

Remember, it is never too late to start exercising and reaping the benefits of an active lifestyle. By creating an exercise routine that suits your needs and preferences, you can enhance your physical and mental well-being, improve longevity, and age well.

3.4 OVERCOMING BARRIERS TO EXERCISE

Exercise is a crucial component of healthy aging. It helps to maintain muscle strength, flexibility, and cardiovascular health, as well as improve mood and cognitive function. However, many individuals face barriers that prevent them from engaging in regular exercise. In this section, we will explore some common barriers to exercise and provide strategies for overcoming them.

3.4.1 Lack of Time

One of the most common barriers to exercise is a perceived lack of time. Many individuals lead busy lives, juggling work, family, and other responsibilities. However, it is important to prioritize exercise for the sake of our long-term health and well-being. Here are some strategies for overcoming the lack of time barrier:

Schedule it in: Treat exercise as an important appointment and schedule it into your daily or weekly routine. Set aside specific time slots for physical activity and stick to them.

Multitask: Look for opportunities to incorporate exercise into your daily activities. For example, take the stairs instead of the elevator, walk or bike to work, or do household chores that require physical effort.

Break it up: If finding a continuous block of time for exercise is challenging, break it up into shorter sessions throughout the day. Even 10 minutes of exercise at a time can be beneficial.

Combine activities: Combine exercise with other activities you enjoy. For example, listen to an audiobook or podcast while walking or jogging, or join a group exercise class to socialize while getting active.

3.4.2 Lack of Motivation

Another common barrier to exercise is a lack of motivation. It can be challenging to find the drive to exercise regularly, especially when faced with fatigue, stress, or other competing priorities. Here are some strategies for overcoming the lack of motivation barrier:

Set goals: Set specific, achievable goals for your exercise routine. Whether it's completing a certain number of workouts per week or improving your endurance, having goals can provide motivation and a sense of accomplishment.

Find your why: Identify the reasons why exercise is important to you. Whether it's improving your health, reducing stress, or increasing your energy levels, reminding yourself of the benefits can help you stay motivated.

Make it enjoyable: Find activities that you genuinely enjoy. Whether it's dancing, swimming, hiking, or playing a sport, engaging in activities that you find fun and enjoyable will make it easier to stay motivated.

Accountability: Find an exercise buddy or join a group or class where you are held accountable for showing up. Having someone to exercise with or a community to support you can provide motivation and make exercise more enjoyable.

3.4.3 Physical Limitations

Physical limitations, such as chronic pain, injuries, or mobility issues, can be significant barriers to exercise. However, it is still possible to engage in physical activity with modifications and adaptations. Here are some strategies for overcoming physical limitations:

Consult a healthcare professional: If you have physical limitations, it is important to consult with a healthcare professional before starting an exercise routine. They can provide guidance on safe and appropriate exercises for your specific condition.

Modify exercises: Work with a qualified fitness professional who can help you modify exercises to accommodate your physical limitations. For example, if you have knee pain, they can suggest low-impact exercises that put less stress on the joints.

Explore alternative activities: If certain types of exercise are not feasible due to physical limitations, explore alternative activities that are more suitable. For example, swimming or water aerobics can be excellent options for individuals with joint pain or limited mobility.

Focus on what you can do: Instead of dwelling on what you can't do, focus on what you can do. Find activities that you enjoy and that are within your physical capabilities. Remember that any form of movement is beneficial for your health.

3.4.4 Lack of Support

Having a support system can greatly enhance your ability to overcome barriers to exercise. Lack of support from family, friends, or the community can make it more challenging to stay motivated and consistent with your exercise routine. Here are some strategies for overcoming the lack of support barrier:

Communicate your goals: Share your exercise goals with your loved ones and explain why they are important to you. By communicating your goals, you can gain their understanding and support.

Find a workout buddy: Find a friend or family member who shares similar exercise goals and become workout buddies. Exercising together can provide motivation, accountability, and make the experience more enjoyable.

Join a fitness community: Join a local fitness group, class, or club where you can connect with like-minded individuals who share similar interests and goals. Being part of a community can provide support, encouragement, and a sense of belonging.

Utilize online resources: If you don't have access to a local fitness community, utilize online resources such as fitness forums, social media groups, or virtual fitness classes. These platforms can provide support, guidance, and motivation from a distance.

By implementing these strategies, you can overcome the barriers that may be preventing you from engaging in regular exercise. Remember, it's never too late to start prioritizing your health and well-being through physical activity.

4. MENTAL HEALTH AND AGING

4.1 MAINTAINING COGNITIVE FUNCTION

As we age, it is natural for our cognitive function to decline to some extent. However, there are steps we can take to maintain and even improve our cognitive abilities as we grow older. In this section, we will explore various strategies and lifestyle choices that can help us maintain cognitive function and promote healthy brain aging.

4.1.1 Engage in Mental Stimulation

One of the most effective ways to maintain cognitive function is to engage in regular mental stimulation. Just like physical exercise keeps our bodies fit, mental exercise keeps our brains sharp. Activities such as reading, puzzles, learning new skills, and playing strategic games can all help stimulate our brains and improve cognitive function.

It is important to challenge ourselves with activities that require problem-solving, critical thinking, and memory recall. This can include activities like crossword puzzles, Sudoku, chess, or learning a new language. By regularly engaging in these activities, we can keep our minds active and enhance our cognitive abilities.

4.1.2 Stay Physically Active

Physical exercise not only benefits our physical health but also plays a crucial role in maintaining cognitive function. Regular exercise increases blood flow to the brain, promotes the growth of new brain cells, and improves memory and cognitive abilities.

Engaging in aerobic exercises like walking, jogging, swimming, or cycling can have a positive impact on cognitive function. Additionally, activities that require coordination and balance, such as yoga or tai chi, can also help improve cognitive abilities.

4.1.3 Follow a Healthy Diet

A healthy diet is essential for maintaining cognitive function. Certain nutrients have been found to support brain health and protect against cognitive decline. Include foods rich in antioxidants, such as fruits and vegetables, to reduce oxidative stress and inflammation in the brain.

Omega-3 fatty acids, found in fatty fish like salmon and sardines, as well as walnuts and flaxseeds, are beneficial for brain health. These healthy fats help reduce inflammation and support the growth and maintenance of brain cells.

Limiting the intake of processed foods, sugary snacks, and saturated fats is also important for brain health. These foods can contribute to inflammation and increase the risk of cognitive decline.

4.1.4 Get Quality Sleep

Sleep plays a vital role in cognitive function and overall brain health. During sleep, the brain consolidates memories, clears out toxins, and restores itself. Chronic sleep deprivation can lead to cognitive impairment and increase the risk of neurodegenerative diseases.

To promote quality sleep, establish a regular sleep routine and create a sleep-friendly environment.

Avoid stimulating activities and electronic devices before bed, and create a calm and comfortable sleep environment. If you are experiencing sleep issues, consult with a healthcare professional for guidance and support.

4.1.5 Manage Stress

Chronic stress can have a negative impact on cognitive function. Prolonged exposure to stress hormones can damage brain cells and impair memory and cognitive abilities. Therefore, it is important to develop effective stress management techniques.

Engaging in activities like meditation, deep breathing exercises, yoga, or spending time in nature can help reduce stress levels. Additionally, maintaining a healthy work-life balance, practicing time management, and seeking social support can also contribute to stress reduction and improved cognitive function.

4.1.6 Stay Socially Active

Maintaining social connections is not only important for our emotional well-being but also for our cognitive health. Engaging in social activities and maintaining strong relationships can help stimulate our brains and reduce the risk of cognitive decline.

Participating in social activities, joining clubs or organizations, volunteering, or simply spending time with loved ones can all contribute to maintaining cognitive function. Social interactions provide mental stimulation, emotional support, and opportunities for learning and growth.

4.1.7 Continual Learning

Never stop learning! Engaging in lifelong learning can help keep our brains active and promote cognitive function. Whether it's taking up a new hobby, enrolling in a course, or attending workshops and seminars, the process of learning stimulates our brains and helps maintain cognitive abilities.

By challenging ourselves to acquire new knowledge and skills, we create new neural connections and enhance our cognitive reserve. This cognitive reserve acts as a buffer against age-related cognitive decline and can help us maintain cognitive function for longer.

Maintaining cognitive function as we age requires a holistic approach that includes mental stimulation, physical exercise, a healthy diet, quality sleep, stress management, social engagement, and continual learning. By implementing these strategies into our daily lives, we can promote healthy brain aging and enjoy a higher quality of life as we grow older.

4.2 Managing Stress and Emotional Well-being

Stress and emotional well-being play a significant role in our overall health and longevity. As we age, it becomes even more crucial to manage stress effectively and prioritize our emotional well-being. Chronic stress can have detrimental effects on our physical and mental health, leading to a higher risk of age-related diseases and a decreased quality of life. In this section, we will explore various strategies to manage stress and enhance emotional well-being, allowing us to age gracefully and maintain optimal health.

4.2.1 Understanding Stress and Its Impact on Aging

Stress is a natural response to challenging situations, and in small doses, it can even be beneficial. However, chronic stress, which occurs when we experience prolonged periods of stress without relief, can have severe consequences for our health. When we are under stress, our bodies release stress hormones like cortisol, which, when constantly elevated, can lead to inflammation, weakened immune function, and an increased risk of chronic diseases such as heart disease, diabetes, and cognitive decline.

As we age, our bodies may become more vulnerable to the negative effects of stress. Our ability to cope with stressors may decrease, and we may be more susceptible to the physical and emotional toll it takes. Therefore, it is essential to develop effective stress management techniques to protect our well-being and promote healthy aging.

4.2.2 Stress Management Techniques for Aging Well

4.2.2.1 Mindfulness and Meditation

Mindfulness and meditation practices have gained significant attention in recent years for their ability to reduce stress and promote emotional well-being. These practices involve focusing our attention on the present moment, cultivating a non-judgmental awareness of our thoughts and feelings. Research has shown that regular mindfulness and meditation practice can lower stress levels, improve mood, and enhance overall mental health.

To incorporate mindfulness into your daily routine, you can start with short meditation sessions of just a few minutes each day. Find a quiet and comfortable space, close your eyes, and focus on your breath or a specific object. Allow your thoughts to come and go without judgment, gently bringing your attention back to the present moment whenever your mind wanders. Over time, you can gradually increase the duration of your meditation sessions and explore different mindfulness techniques that resonate with you.

4.2.2.2 Physical Activity and Exercise

Engaging in regular physical activity and exercise is not only beneficial for our physical health but also plays a crucial role in managing stress and promoting emotional well-being. Exercise releases endorphins, which are natural mood-boosting chemicals in the brain. It can also help reduce anxiety, improve sleep quality, and enhance self-esteem.

Incorporating exercise into your daily routine doesn't have to be complicated or time-consuming. Aim for at least 150 minutes of moderate-intensity aerobic activity, such as brisk walking or cycling, per week. Additionally, include strength training exercises at least twice a week to maintain muscle mass and bone density. Find activities that you enjoy and make them a regular part of your schedule. Whether it's dancing, swimming, gardening, or practicing yoga, find what brings you joy and helps you manage stress effectively.

4.2.2.3 Social Connections and Support

Maintaining strong social connections and

seeking support from loved ones is essential for managing stress and promoting emotional well-being. As we age, our social networks may change, and it becomes even more crucial to nurture existing relationships and cultivate new ones. Spending time with family and friends, participating in group activities, and joining clubs or organizations that align with your interests can provide a sense of belonging and support.

If you find yourself feeling isolated or lacking social connections, consider reaching out to community organizations or support groups that cater to older adults. Volunteering can also be a great way to connect with others while making a positive impact in your community. Remember, it's never too late to forge new friendships and build a strong support system.

4.2.2.4 Self-Care and Relaxation Techniques

Practicing self-care and incorporating relaxation techniques into your daily routine can significantly contribute to managing stress and enhancing emotional well-being. Self-care involves prioritizing activities that bring you joy, relaxation, and rejuvenation. It can be as simple as taking a warm bath, reading a book, listening to music, or engaging in a hobby you love.

In addition to self-care, relaxation techniques such as deep breathing exercises, progressive muscle relaxation, and aromatherapy can help calm the mind and reduce stress levels. Experiment with different techniques and find what works best for you. Incorporating these practices into your daily life can provide a sense of balance and help you navigate the challenges of aging with greater ease.

4.2.3 Seeking Professional Help

Sometimes, managing stress and emotional well-being may require professional help. If you find that stress is significantly impacting your daily life, relationships, or overall well-being, it is essential to seek support from a healthcare professional or mental health specialist. They can provide guidance, offer coping strategies, and help you navigate any underlying issues contributing to your stress.

Remember, managing stress and emotional well-being is a lifelong journey. It requires consistent effort and a commitment to self-care. By implementing these strategies and seeking support when needed, you can effectively manage stress, enhance emotional well-being, and age well, allowing you to enjoy a long and fulfilling life.

4.3 SOCIAL CONNECTIONS AND AGING

Social connections play a vital role in our overall

well-being, and this is especially true as we age. Maintaining strong social connections can have a significant impact on our physical and mental health, as well as our longevity. In this section, we will explore the importance of social connections in aging and provide strategies for fostering and maintaining meaningful relationships.

4.3.1 The Impact of Social Connections on Aging

Research has consistently shown that social connections have a profound effect on our health and well-being as we age. Strong social ties have been linked to a reduced risk of chronic diseases, such as heart disease, stroke, and Alzheimer's disease. Additionally, individuals with robust social networks tend to have lower levels of stress, depression, and anxiety.

One reason social connections are so beneficial is that they provide a sense of belonging and purpose. When we have meaningful relationships, we feel supported, valued, and understood. This sense of belonging can boost our self-esteem and overall life satisfaction. Furthermore, social connections can provide a support system during challenging times, helping us cope with stress and adversity.

4.3.2 Building and Maintaining Social

Connections

Building and maintaining social connections requires effort and intentionality, but the rewards are well worth it. Here are some strategies to help you foster and maintain meaningful relationships as you age:

4.3.2.1 Cultivate Existing Relationships

Start by nurturing the relationships you already have. Reach out to old friends, family members, or acquaintances you haven't seen in a while. Schedule regular catch-ups, whether it's meeting for coffee, going for a walk, or simply having a phone call. By investing time and energy into these relationships, you can strengthen the bond and create lasting connections.

4.3.2.2 Join Social Groups and Clubs

Engaging in social activities is an excellent way to meet new people and expand your social circle. Consider joining clubs, community organizations, or hobby groups that align with your interests. This can provide opportunities to connect with like-minded individuals and form new friendships. Whether it's a book club, a gardening group, or a volunteer organization, finding activities that bring you joy can also lead to meaningful social connections.

4.3.2.3 Embrace Technology

Technology has made it easier than ever to stay

connected with others, regardless of physical distance. Utilize social media platforms, video calls, and messaging apps to keep in touch with friends and family members who may live far away. Virtual gatherings and online communities can also provide a sense of belonging and connection. However, it's important to strike a balance and not rely solely on virtual interactions. Face-to-face interactions are still crucial for building deep and meaningful relationships.

4.3.2.4 Volunteer and Give Back

Engaging in volunteer work not only benefits the community but also provides an opportunity to connect with others who share similar values. Look for local organizations or charities that align with your interests and offer your time and skills. Volunteering can not only provide a sense of purpose and fulfillment but also introduce you to new people and expand your social network.

4.3.2.5 Seek Support Groups

If you are facing specific challenges or health conditions, consider joining support groups. These groups provide a safe space to share experiences, receive emotional support, and learn from others who may be going through similar situations. Whether it's a support group for caregivers, individuals with chronic illnesses, or those experiencing grief, these groups can offer a sense of understanding and camaraderie.

4.3.3 The Role of Intergenerational Connections

Intergenerational connections, or relationships between different age groups, are particularly valuable for aging individuals. These connections provide opportunities for learning, growth, and mutual support. Here are some ways to foster intergenerational connections:

4.3.3.1 Spend Time with Family

Make an effort to spend quality time with your children, grandchildren, or other younger family members. Engage in activities that allow for meaningful interactions, such as cooking together, playing games, or sharing stories. These interactions not only strengthen family bonds but also provide opportunities for learning and creating lasting memories.

4.3.3.2 Volunteer or Mentor

Consider volunteering or mentoring programs that connect older adults with younger individuals. This can be a rewarding experience that allows you to share your wisdom, skills, and life experiences with the younger generation. Mentoring relationships can be mutually beneficial, providing both parties with valuable insights and support.

4.3.3.3 Participate in Intergenerational Programs

Look for intergenerational programs in your community that bring different age groups together. These programs may include activities such as art classes, community gardening, or intergenerational sports teams. Participating in these programs can foster understanding, empathy, and connection between generations.

4.3.4 The Importance of Quality Relationships

While it's essential to have a wide social network, the quality of your relationships is equally important. Focus on cultivating deep and meaningful connections with a few individuals rather than having a large number of superficial relationships. Quality relationships provide emotional support, companionship, and a sense of belonging that can significantly impact your well-being as you age.

Conclusion

Social connections are a fundamental aspect of aging well. By investing in and nurturing meaningful relationships, you can enhance your physical and mental health, increase your longevity, and experience a greater sense of fulfillment and happiness. Whether it's through existing relationships, social groups, technology, volunteering, or intergenerational connections, there are numerous opportunities to foster and maintain social connections as you age. Embrace the power of social connections and enjoy the benefits they bring to your overall well-being.

4.4 MENTAL HEALTH STRATEGIES FOR LONGEVITY

Mental health plays a crucial role in our overall well-being and is an essential component of aging well. As we age, it becomes increasingly important to prioritize our mental health and take proactive steps to maintain cognitive function, manage stress, and foster emotional well-being. In this section, we will explore various strategies and techniques that can help promote mental health and longevity.

4.4.1 Cognitive Stimulation

One of the key aspects of maintaining mental health as we age is to engage in activities that stimulate our cognitive abilities. Just like physical exercise keeps our bodies fit, cognitive stimulation exercises keep our minds sharp. These exercises can include puzzles, brain games, reading, learning a new skill or language, and engaging in intellectually stimulating conversations. By challenging our brains regularly, we can enhance our cognitive function and reduce the risk of cognitive decline and age-related conditions such as dementia.

4.4.2 Stress Management

Stress can have a significant impact on our mental health and overall well-being. Chronic stress can contribute to the development of various health issues, including cardiovascular problems, weakened immune system, and mental health disorders. Therefore, it is crucial to develop effective stress management techniques to mitigate its negative effects.

One effective strategy for managing stress is practicing relaxation techniques such as deep breathing exercises, meditation, and mindfulness. These techniques help calm the mind, reduce anxiety, and promote a sense of inner peace. Additionally, engaging in regular physical exercise, maintaining a healthy diet, and getting enough sleep can also help reduce stress levels.

4.4.3 Emotional Well-being

Emotional well-being is closely linked to mental health and plays a vital role in our overall happiness and quality of life. As we age, it is essential to pay attention to our emotional needs and take steps to nurture positive emotions and manage negative ones.

One effective strategy for promoting emotional well-being is practicing gratitude. Taking time each day to reflect on the things we are grateful for can help shift our focus towards positivity and increase feelings of contentment. Additionally, engaging in activities that bring joy and fulfillment, such as hobbies, spending time with loved ones, and pursuing meaningful goals, can contribute to emotional well-being.

4.4.4 Social Connections

Maintaining strong social connections is crucial for our mental health and longevity. As we age, it is common for social networks to shrink due to various factors such as retirement, loss of loved ones, or physical limitations. However, it is essential to actively seek out and nurture social connections to combat feelings of loneliness and isolation.

Engaging in social activities, joining clubs or community groups, volunteering, and staying connected with family and friends can help foster a sense of belonging and provide opportunities for meaningful social interactions. Additionally, technology can also be a valuable tool for staying connected with loved ones, especially for those who may have limited mobility or live far away.

4.4.5 Seeking Professional Help

Sometimes, despite our best efforts, we may find ourselves struggling with mental health issues that require professional help. It is important to recognize when we need assistance and not hesitate to seek help from mental health professionals.

Therapy or counseling can provide a safe and supportive environment to explore and address any underlying mental health concerns. A trained therapist can offer guidance, coping strategies, and tools to manage stress, anxiety, depression, or other mental health conditions. Seeking professional help is a sign of strength and a proactive step towards maintaining optimal mental health and well-being.

4.4.6 Self-Care and Mindfulness

Practicing self-care and mindfulness is essential for maintaining mental health and longevity. Self-care involves prioritizing our own well-being and taking time to engage in activities that bring us joy, relaxation, and rejuvenation. This can include activities such as taking a bath, practicing yoga or meditation, reading a book, or spending time in nature.

Mindfulness, on the other hand, involves being fully present in the moment and cultivating a non-judgmental awareness of our thoughts, feelings, and sensations. By practicing mindfulness, we can reduce stress, enhance self-awareness, and improve our overall mental well-being.

4.4.7 Maintaining a Positive Outlook

Maintaining a positive outlook on life can have a profound impact on our mental health and overall well-being. Optimism and positive thinking can help reduce stress, improve resilience, and enhance our ability to cope with challenges that come with aging.

Cultivating a positive mindset involves reframing negative thoughts, focusing on the present moment, and practicing gratitude. By consciously choosing to see the silver lining in difficult situations and adopting a growth mindset, we can cultivate a positive outlook that contributes to our mental health and longevity.

Prioritizing mental health is crucial for aging well and maintaining overall well-being. By engaging in cognitive stimulation exercises, managing stress, nurturing emotional well-being, fostering social connections, seeking professional help when needed, practicing self-care and mindfulness, and maintaining a positive outlook, we can promote mental health and longevity. Remember, it is never too late to start implementing these strategies and taking proactive steps towards a mentally healthy and fulfilling life as we age.

5. SLEEP AND AGING

5.1 THE IMPORTANCE OF SLEEP FOR AGING WELL

Sleep is a fundamental aspect of our overall health and well-being, and it becomes even more crucial as we age. Adequate sleep is essential for maintaining physical and mental health, and it plays a vital role in the aging process. In this section, we will explore the importance of sleep for aging well and discuss strategies to improve sleep quality.

5.1.1 The Role of Sleep in Aging

Sleep is a restorative process that allows our bodies and minds to recharge and repair. It is during sleep that our bodies undergo essential processes such as tissue repair, hormone regulation, and memory consolidation. As we age, the quality and quantity of our sleep can be affected by various factors, including changes in our sleep patterns and the presence of age-related conditions.

5.1.2 The Impact of Sleep on Physical Health

Adequate sleep is crucial for maintaining optimal physical health as we age. Research has shown that insufficient sleep can contribute to a range of health issues, including obesity, diabetes, cardiovascular disease, and weakened immune function. Lack of sleep can also impair our ability to recover from illness or injury, making it even more important to prioritize quality sleep as we get older.

5.1.3 The Impact of Sleep on Mental Health

In addition to its effects on physical health, sleep also plays a significant role in our mental well-being. Sufficient sleep is essential for cognitive function, memory consolidation, and emotional regulation. As we age, the risk of developing cognitive decline and neurodegenerative disorders such as Alzheimer's disease increases. Research suggests that poor sleep quality and duration may contribute to the development of these conditions. By prioritizing sleep, we can potentially reduce the risk of cognitive decline and promote better mental health as we age.

Sleep is a vital component of healthy aging. By understanding the importance of sleep and implementing strategies to improve sleep quality, we can enhance our physical and mental well-being as we age. Prioritizing sleep and addressing any sleep-related issues can contribute to a higher quality of life and promote longevity.

5.2 COMMON SLEEP ISSUES IN AGING

As we age, our sleep patterns and needs change. It is not uncommon for older adults to experience sleep issues that can affect their overall health and well-being. In this section, we will explore some of the common sleep issues that occur with aging and discuss strategies for improving sleep quality.

5.2.1 Insomnia

Insomnia is a common sleep disorder that affects people of all ages, but it becomes more prevalent as we get older. Older adults may have difficulty falling asleep, staying asleep, or waking up too early in the morning. Insomnia can be caused by a variety of factors, including stress, anxiety, medication side effects, and underlying health conditions.

To improve sleep quality and manage insomnia, it is important to establish a regular sleep routine. This includes going to bed and waking up at the same time every day, even on weekends. Creating a relaxing bedtime routine can also help signal to your body that it is time to sleep. This may involve activities such as reading a book, taking a warm bath, or practicing relaxation techniques like deep breathing or meditation.

Avoiding stimulants such as caffeine and nicotine close to bedtime is also important. These substances can interfere with your ability to fall asleep and stay asleep. It is also advisable to limit daytime napping, as excessive napping can disrupt your sleep-wake cycle.

If insomnia persists despite these strategies, it may be helpful to consult with a healthcare professional. They can assess your sleep patterns, identify any underlying causes, and recommend appropriate treatment options such as cognitive-behavioral therapy for insomnia (CBT-I) or medication if necessary.

5.2.2 Sleep Apnea

Sleep apnea is a sleep disorder characterized by pauses in breathing or shallow breaths during sleep. It is more common in older adults and can have serious health consequences if left untreated. Sleep apnea can lead to daytime sleepiness, fatigue, and an increased risk of cardiovascular problems.

If you suspect you may have sleep apnea, it is important to seek medical attention. A healthcare professional can conduct a sleep study to diagnose the condition and recommend appropriate treatment options. Continuous positive airway pressure (CPAP) therapy is a common treatment for sleep apnea, which involves wearing a mask that delivers a constant flow of air to keep the airway open during sleep.

In addition to medical treatment, there are lifestyle changes that can help manage sleep apnea. Maintaining a healthy weight, avoiding alcohol and sedatives before bed, and sleeping on your side instead of your back can all contribute to improved sleep quality for individuals with sleep apnea.

5.2.3 Restless Legs Syndrome (RLS)

Restless Legs Syndrome (RLS) is a neurological disorder characterized by an irresistible urge to move the legs, often accompanied by uncomfortable sensations such as tingling or crawling. RLS symptoms tend to worsen during periods of rest or inactivity, making it difficult to fall asleep or stay asleep.

If you experience symptoms of RLS, it is important to consult with a healthcare professional for proper diagnosis and management. Treatment options for RLS may include lifestyle changes, such as regular exercise and avoiding triggers like caffeine and nicotine. Medications can also be prescribed to alleviate symptoms and improve sleep quality.

5.2.4 Periodic Limb Movement Disorder (PLMD)

Periodic Limb Movement Disorder (PLMD) is a sleep disorder characterized by repetitive movements of the legs or arms during sleep. These movements can disrupt sleep and lead to daytime sleepiness and fatigue. PLMD is more common in older adults and can be associated with other conditions such as restless legs syndrome or sleep apnea.

Treatment for PLMD may involve addressing any underlying conditions, such as treating sleep apnea or managing restless legs syndrome. Medications can also be prescribed to reduce the frequency and intensity of limb movements during sleep.

5.2.5 Other Sleep Issues

In addition to the sleep issues mentioned above,

older adults may also experience other common sleep problems such as:

Nocturia: The need to wake up frequently during the night to urinate. This can disrupt sleep and lead to daytime fatigue. Managing fluid intake, especially in the evening, and addressing any underlying medical conditions can help alleviate nocturia.

Shifted Sleep-Wake Cycle: Older adults may find that their sleep-wake cycle shifts, causing them to feel sleepy earlier in the evening and wake up earlier in the morning. Establishing a consistent sleep schedule and exposing yourself to natural light during the day can help regulate your sleep-wake cycle.

Age-Related Changes in Sleep Architecture: As we age, there are changes in the structure and quality of our sleep. Older adults may experience lighter sleep, more frequent awakenings, and less time spent in deep sleep or REM sleep. While these changes are a normal part of aging, practicing good sleep hygiene and implementing strategies to improve sleep quality can help mitigate their effects.

Sleep issues are common in aging adults, but they can be managed with the right strategies and interventions. Establishing a regular sleep routine, addressing underlying health conditions, and seeking medical advice when necessary are all important steps in improving sleep quality and promoting overall well-being.

5.3 IMPROVING SLEEP QUALITY

Sleep is an essential component of overall health and well-being, and it becomes even more crucial as we age. Unfortunately, many older adults struggle with sleep issues, such as insomnia, sleep fragmentation, and difficulty staying asleep. These sleep disturbances can have a significant impact on our physical and mental health, leading to increased risk of chronic conditions, cognitive decline, and reduced quality of life. However, there are several strategies that can help improve sleep quality and promote healthy aging.

5.3.1 Establish a Consistent Sleep Schedule

One of the most effective ways to improve sleep quality is to establish a consistent sleep schedule. Going to bed and waking up at the same time every day helps regulate our body's internal clock, known as the circadian rhythm. This internal clock plays a crucial role in regulating sleep-wake cycles and maintaining optimal sleep quality. By sticking to a regular sleep schedule, we can train our bodies to fall asleep faster and stay asleep throughout the night.

5.3.2 Create a Relaxing Bedtime Routine

Creating a relaxing bedtime routine can signal to

our bodies that it's time to wind down and prepare for sleep. Engaging in calming activities before bed can help reduce stress and promote relaxation. Some effective bedtime routine practices include taking a warm bath, practicing deep breathing exercises, reading a book, or listening to soothing music. It's important to avoid stimulating activities, such as using electronic devices or engaging in intense exercise, close to bedtime, as they can interfere with sleep.

5.3.3 Create a Sleep-Friendly Environment

The environment in which we sleep can greatly impact the quality of our sleep. It's essential to create a sleep-friendly environment that is conducive to relaxation and restfulness. Keep your bedroom cool, dark, and quiet. Consider using blackout curtains, earplugs, or a white noise machine to block out any external disturbances. Additionally, invest in a comfortable mattress and pillows that provide adequate support for your body. Creating a peaceful and comfortable sleep environment can significantly improve sleep quality.

5.3.4 Limit Exposure to Electronic Devices

The blue light emitted by electronic devices, such as smartphones, tablets, and computers, can interfere with our sleep-wake cycles. Exposure to blue light in the evening can suppress the production of melatonin, a hormone that regulates sleep. To improve sleep quality, it's important to limit exposure to electronic devices, especially in the hours leading up to bedtime. Consider implementing a "digital detox" by turning off electronic devices at least an hour before bed and engaging in relaxing activities instead.

5.3.5 Manage Stress and Anxiety

Stress and anxiety can significantly impact sleep quality, making it difficult to fall asleep and stay asleep. It's important to develop effective stress management techniques to promote better sleep. Engaging in relaxation techniques, such as meditation, deep breathing exercises, or yoga, can help reduce stress and promote a sense of calm before bed. Additionally, consider addressing any underlying sources of stress or anxiety through therapy or counseling. By managing stress and anxiety effectively, we can improve sleep quality and overall well-being.

5.3.6 Regular Physical Activity

Regular physical activity has numerous benefits for sleep quality and overall health. Engaging in moderate-intensity exercise, such as walking, swimming, or cycling, can help regulate sleep patterns and promote better sleep. However, it's important to time exercise appropriately.

Exercising too close to bedtime can have a stimulating effect on the body, making it difficult to fall asleep. Aim to finish your workout at least a few hours before bed to allow your body to wind down and prepare for sleep.

5.3.7 Limit Caffeine and Alcohol Intake

Caffeine and alcohol can have a significant impact on sleep quality. Caffeine is a stimulant that can interfere with falling asleep and staying asleep. It's important to limit caffeine intake, especially in the afternoon and evening. Be mindful of hidden sources of caffeine, such as chocolate and certain medications. Similarly, while alcohol may initially make you feel drowsy, it can disrupt the later stages of sleep, leading to poor sleep quality. It's best to avoid alcohol close to bedtime to promote better sleep.

5.3.8 Seek Professional Help if Needed

If you have tried various strategies to improve sleep quality and are still experiencing significant sleep disturbances, it may be beneficial to seek professional help. A healthcare provider or sleep specialist can evaluate your sleep patterns, identify any underlying sleep disorders, and recommend appropriate treatment options. They may suggest techniques such as cognitive-behavioral therapy for insomnia (CBT-I) or prescribe medications if necessary. Remember, it's essential to address sleep issues to promote healthy aging and overall well-being.

Improving sleep quality is a vital aspect of aging well. By implementing these strategies and making sleep a priority, you can enhance your overall health, cognitive function, and quality of life as you age. Remember, everyone's sleep needs are different, so it's important to find what works best for you and establish healthy sleep habits that support your individual needs.

5.4 CREATING A HEALTHY SLEEP ROUTINE

Sleep is an essential component of our overall health and well-being, and it becomes even more crucial as we age. A good night's sleep not only helps us feel refreshed and energized but also plays a vital role in maintaining our physical and mental health. In this section, we will explore the importance of creating a healthy sleep routine and provide practical tips for improving the quality of your sleep as you age.

5.4.1 Understanding the Importance of Sleep

Sleep is a natural process that allows our bodies and minds to rest, repair, and rejuvenate. It is during sleep that our bodies heal and regenerate cells, strengthen the immune system, and consolidate memories. Adequate sleep is essential for maintaining optimal cognitive function, emotional well-being, and overall physical health.

As we age, our sleep patterns tend to change. Older adults may experience difficulty falling asleep, staying asleep throughout the night, or waking up too early. These changes can be attributed to various factors, including hormonal changes, medical conditions, medications, and lifestyle factors. However, it is important to note that poor sleep is not an inevitable part of aging and can be improved with the right sleep routine.

5.4.2 Establishing a Consistent Sleep Schedule

One of the key strategies for creating a healthy sleep routine is to establish a consistent sleep schedule. Going to bed and waking up at the same time every day, even on weekends, helps regulate your body's internal clock and promotes better sleep quality. Aim for a sleep duration of 7-9 hours per night, as recommended by sleep experts.

To establish a consistent sleep schedule, start by determining the ideal bedtime that allows you to get enough sleep and wake up feeling refreshed. Gradually adjust your bedtime and wake-up time until you reach your desired schedule. Be patient with the process, as it may take a few weeks for your body to adjust to the new routine.

5.4.3 Creating a Relaxing Bedtime Routine

A relaxing bedtime routine can signal to your body that it's time to wind down and prepare for sleep. Engaging in calming activities before bed can help promote relaxation and improve sleep quality. Consider incorporating the following practices into your bedtime routine:

Limit screen time: The blue light emitted by electronic devices can interfere with your sleep-wake cycle. Avoid using electronic devices such as smartphones, tablets, and computers at least an hour before bed.

Create a peaceful environment: Make your bedroom a sleep-friendly environment by keeping it cool, dark, and quiet. Use blackout curtains or an eye mask to block out any unwanted light, and consider using earplugs or a white noise machine to mask any disruptive sounds.

Engage in relaxation techniques: Practice relaxation techniques such as deep breathing, meditation, or gentle stretching before bed. These activities can help calm your mind and prepare your body for sleep.

Avoid stimulating substances: Limit your intake of caffeine, nicotine, and alcohol, as these substances can interfere with your sleep. It's best to avoid consuming them close to bedtime.

5.4.4 Creating a Comfortable Sleep Environment

The quality of your sleep environment can significantly impact your sleep quality. Creating a comfortable and conducive sleep environment can help you fall asleep faster and stay asleep throughout the night. Consider the following tips:

Invest in a supportive mattress and pillows: A comfortable mattress and pillows that provide adequate support for your body can make a significant difference in your sleep quality. Choose a mattress and pillows that suit your preferences and ensure proper spinal alignment.

Choose breathable bedding: Opt for breathable bedding materials such as cotton or bamboo, which can help regulate your body temperature and prevent overheating during sleep.

Keep your bedroom clutter-free: A clutter-free bedroom can promote a sense of calm and relaxation. Keep your bedroom clean and organized to create a peaceful sleep environment.

Manage noise and light: Use earplugs, a white noise machine, or a fan to mask any disruptive sounds. Consider using blackout curtains or an eye mask to block out any unwanted light.

5.4.5 Managing Sleep Disorders and Seeking Professional Help

If you continue to experience persistent sleep issues despite implementing healthy sleep habits, it may be beneficial to consult a healthcare professional. Sleep disorders such as insomnia, sleep apnea, restless leg syndrome, and narcolepsy can significantly impact your sleep quality and overall well-being. A healthcare professional can help diagnose and treat these conditions, providing you with personalized strategies to improve your sleep.

Creating a healthy sleep routine is essential for aging well. By establishing a consistent sleep schedule, engaging in a relaxing bedtime routine, creating a comfortable sleep environment, and seeking professional help when needed, you can improve the quality of your sleep and enhance your overall health and well-being as you age. Remember, a good night's sleep is a vital component of your longevity blueprint.

6. PREVENTING AGE-RELATED DISEASES

6.1 UNDERSTANDING AGE-RELATED DISEASES

As we age, our bodies undergo various changes that can increase the risk of developing age-related diseases. Understanding these diseases and their underlying causes is crucial for taking proactive steps to prevent and manage them. In this section, we will explore the most common age-related diseases, their risk factors, and strategies for reducing their impact on our health.

6.1.1 Cardiovascular Diseases

Cardiovascular diseases, including heart disease

and stroke, are leading causes of death and disability among older adults. These diseases occur when there is a buildup of plaque in the arteries, leading to reduced blood flow to the heart or brain. Several factors contribute to the development of cardiovascular diseases, including high blood pressure, high cholesterol levels, smoking, obesity, and a sedentary lifestyle.

To prevent heart disease and stroke, it is essential to adopt a heart-healthy lifestyle. This includes maintaining a balanced diet rich in fruits, vegetables, whole grains, and lean proteins. Regular exercise, such as aerobic activities and strength training, can help improve cardiovascular health. Managing stress, quitting smoking, and maintaining a healthy weight are also crucial for reducing the risk of cardiovascular diseases.

6.1.2 Cancer

Cancer is another significant age-related disease that affects millions of people worldwide. It occurs when abnormal cells divide and grow uncontrollably, forming tumors. Age is a significant risk factor for cancer, with the risk increasing as we get older. Other factors that contribute to the development of cancer include exposure to carcinogens, genetic predisposition, and lifestyle choices such as smoking, poor diet, and lack of physical activity.

Reducing the risk of cancer involves adopting a healthy lifestyle and taking preventive measures. Eating a diet rich in fruits, vegetables, whole grains, and lean proteins can help protect against certain types of cancer. Avoiding tobacco products and limiting alcohol consumption are also essential for reducing the risk. Regular screenings and early detection can significantly improve the chances of successful treatment.

6.1.3 Chronic Conditions

Chronic conditions such as diabetes, arthritis, and osteoporosis are prevalent among older adults. These conditions can significantly impact quality of life and increase the risk of disability. Chronic conditions often develop due to a combination of genetic factors, lifestyle choices, and age-related changes in the body.

Managing chronic conditions involves a multidimensional approach. It is crucial to work closely with healthcare professionals to develop a personalized treatment plan. This may include medication, physical therapy, dietary changes, and lifestyle modifications. Regular exercise, maintaining a healthy weight, and managing stress can also help reduce the impact of chronic conditions on overall health.

6.1.4 Neurodegenerative Diseases

Neurodegenerative diseases, such as Alzheimer's and Parkinson's disease, are characterized by the progressive degeneration of nerve cells in the brain. These diseases can significantly impact cognitive function, mobility, and overall well-being. While the exact causes of neurodegenerative diseases are not fully understood, age, genetics, and environmental factors are believed to play a role.

Preventing neurodegenerative diseases involves adopting a brain-healthy lifestyle. Regular exercise, a balanced diet, and mental stimulation can help protect against cognitive decline. Engaging in activities that challenge the brain, such as puzzles, reading, and learning new skills, can also promote brain health. Additionally, managing chronic conditions, maintaining social connections, and getting quality sleep are essential for reducing the risk of neurodegenerative diseases.

6.1.5 Strategies for Prevention

Preventing age-related diseases requires a holistic approach that addresses various aspects of health and well-being. Here are some strategies to consider:

Maintain a healthy lifestyle: Adopt a balanced

diet, engage in regular physical activity, manage stress, and avoid harmful habits such as smoking and excessive alcohol consumption.

Regular health screenings: Stay up to date with recommended screenings for conditions such as cancer, heart disease, and diabetes. Early detection can significantly improve treatment outcomes.

Manage chronic conditions: Work closely with healthcare professionals to develop a personalized treatment plan for managing chronic conditions and minimizing their impact on overall health.

Stay mentally and socially active: Engage in activities that challenge the brain, maintain social connections, and seek opportunities for personal growth and learning.

Get quality sleep: Establish a healthy sleep routine and address any sleep issues promptly. Quality sleep is essential for overall health and well-being.

By understanding age-related diseases and implementing preventive strategies, we can significantly improve our chances of aging well and maintaining a high quality of life. It is never too late to start taking proactive steps towards a healthier future.

6.2 PREVENTING HEART DISEASE AND

STROKE

Heart disease and stroke are two of the leading causes of death worldwide, and they become more prevalent as we age. However, the good news is that many cases of heart disease and stroke can be prevented through lifestyle changes and proactive measures. In this section, we will explore the key strategies for preventing heart disease and stroke, allowing you to take control of your cardiovascular health and promote longevity.

6.2.1 Understanding Heart Disease

Before we delve into prevention strategies, it is essential to understand what heart disease entails. Heart disease refers to a range of conditions that affect the heart and blood vessels, including coronary artery disease, heart failure, and arrhythmias. These conditions can lead to serious complications, such as heart attacks and strokes.

6.2.2 The Role of Lifestyle in Heart Disease Prevention

Lifestyle factors play a significant role in the development and prevention of heart disease. By adopting healthy habits, you can significantly reduce your risk of developing heart disease and stroke. Here are some key lifestyle factors to consider:

6.2.2.1 Healthy Eating Habits

A nutritious diet is crucial for maintaining a healthy heart. Focus on consuming a variety of fruits, vegetables, whole grains, lean proteins, and healthy fats. Limit your intake of saturated and trans fats, sodium, and added sugars. Incorporating heart-healthy foods, such as fatty fish, nuts, and olive oil, can provide additional benefits.

6.2.2.2 Regular Physical Activity

Engaging in regular physical activity is vital for cardiovascular health. Aim for at least 150 minutes of moderate-intensity aerobic exercise or 75 minutes of vigorous-intensity exercise each week. Additionally, include strength training exercises to improve muscle strength and endurance. Find activities you enjoy, such as walking, swimming, or cycling, and make them a part of your routine.

6.2.2.3 Maintaining a Healthy Weight

Excess weight puts strain on the heart and increases the risk of heart disease. By maintaining a healthy weight, you can reduce this risk significantly. Focus on achieving a balance between a nutritious diet and regular physical activity to achieve and maintain a healthy weight.

6.2.2.4 Managing Stress

Chronic stress can contribute to the development of heart disease. Implement stress management techniques such as deep breathing exercises, meditation, yoga, or engaging in hobbies and activities that bring you joy. Prioritizing self-care and finding healthy ways to cope with stress can have a positive impact on your heart health.

6.2.2.5 Avoiding Tobacco and Limiting Alcohol

Smoking is a significant risk factor for heart disease and stroke. If you smoke, seek support to quit smoking and avoid exposure to secondhand smoke. Additionally, limit your alcohol consumption to moderate levels. Excessive alcohol intake can increase blood pressure and contribute to heart disease.

6.2.3 Regular Health Check-ups

Regular health check-ups are essential for monitoring your cardiovascular health and detecting any potential issues early on. Schedule regular appointments with your healthcare provider to assess your blood pressure, cholesterol levels, and overall heart health. By identifying and addressing any risk factors or abnormalities promptly, you can take proactive steps to prevent heart disease and stroke.

6.2.4 Managing Chronic Conditions

Chronic conditions such as diabetes, high blood

pressure, and high cholesterol significantly increase the risk of heart disease and stroke. If you have any of these conditions, it is crucial to work closely with your healthcare provider to manage them effectively. Follow your prescribed treatment plan, take medications as directed, and make necessary lifestyle modifications to keep these conditions under control.

6.2.5 Promoting Heart-Healthy Habits in Daily Life

In addition to the strategies mentioned above, there are several other habits you can incorporate into your daily life to promote heart health:

- Get an adequate amount of sleep each night, aiming for 7-8 hours of quality sleep.
- Stay hydrated by drinking plenty of water throughout the day.
- Limit your intake of processed foods, sugary beverages, and unhealthy snacks.
- Incorporate stress-reducing activities into your routine, such as spending time in nature, practicing mindfulness, or engaging in hobbies you enjoy.
- Stay socially connected and maintain strong relationships with family and friends.

By adopting these habits and making them a part of your daily life, you can significantly reduce your risk of heart disease and stroke, promoting a long and healthy life.

6.3 REDUCING THE RISK OF CANCER

Cancer is a complex and multifaceted disease that affects millions of people worldwide. It is characterized by the uncontrolled growth and spread of abnormal cells in the body. As we age, the risk of developing cancer increases, making it crucial to take proactive steps to reduce this risk. While there is no guaranteed way to prevent cancer, there are several strategies that can significantly lower the likelihood of developing the disease. In this section, we will explore these strategies and provide practical tips for reducing the risk of cancer as we age.

6.3.1 Maintain a Healthy Weight

Maintaining a healthy weight is one of the most important factors in reducing the risk of cancer. Obesity has been linked to an increased risk of several types of cancer, including breast, colorectal, and prostate cancer. Excess body fat can lead to chronic inflammation, hormonal imbalances, and insulin resistance, all of which can promote the development and progression of cancer.

To maintain a healthy weight, it is essential to follow a balanced diet and engage in regular physical activity. Focus on consuming a variety of nutrient-dense foods, such as fruits, vegetables, whole grains, and lean proteins. Limit the intake of processed foods, sugary beverages, and high-fat foods. Additionally, aim to engage in at least 150 minutes of moderate-intensity aerobic exercise or 75 minutes of vigorous-intensity exercise per week. Incorporating strength training exercises can also help build and maintain muscle mass, which is important for overall health and metabolism.

6.3.2 Adopt a Healthy Diet

A healthy diet plays a crucial role in reducing the risk of cancer. Certain foods and nutrients have been shown to have protective effects against cancer, while others may increase the risk. To lower your risk of cancer, consider the following dietary recommendations:

Eat a variety of fruits and vegetables: Fruits and vegetables are rich in vitamins, minerals, and antioxidants that help protect against cancer. Aim to include a colorful array of fruits and vegetables in your diet, as different colors indicate different beneficial compounds.

Choose whole grains: Whole grains, such as brown rice, quinoa, and whole wheat bread, are high in fiber and other nutrients that can help reduce the risk of colorectal cancer.

Limit red and processed meats: Consumption of

red and processed meats has been linked to an increased risk of colorectal and other types of cancer. Opt for lean sources of protein, such as poultry, fish, beans, and legumes.

Reduce alcohol consumption: Excessive alcohol consumption has been associated with an increased risk of several types of cancer, including breast, liver, and colorectal cancer. If you choose to drink alcohol, do so in moderation, which means up to one drink per day for women and up to two drinks per day for men.

Avoid sugary drinks and processed foods: High intake of sugary drinks and processed foods has been linked to an increased risk of obesity, which is a risk factor for several types of cancer. Opt for water, herbal tea, or unsweetened beverages, and choose whole, unprocessed foods whenever possible.

6.3.3 Quit Smoking

Smoking is the leading cause of preventable cancer deaths worldwide. It is responsible for approximately one-third of all cancer-related deaths. Quitting smoking is one of the most effective ways to reduce the risk of cancer and improve overall health. Even if you have been smoking for many years, quitting can still provide significant benefits.

When you quit smoking, your risk of developing various types of cancer, including lung, bladder, and pancreatic cancer, decreases over time. Additionally, quitting smoking can improve lung function, reduce the risk of heart disease, and enhance overall quality of life. If you need help quitting, consider reaching out to healthcare professionals or support groups that specialize in smoking cessation.

6.3.4 Protect Yourself from the Sun

Excessive exposure to ultraviolet (UV) radiation from the sun or tanning beds is a major risk factor for skin cancer, including melanoma, the deadliest form of skin cancer. To protect yourself from the sun and reduce the risk of skin cancer:

Seek shade: Limit your time in the sun, especially between 10 a.m. and 4 p.m., when the sun's rays are the strongest.

Wear protective clothing: Cover your skin with long-sleeved shirts, pants, and wide-brimmed hats. Choose clothing with a tight weave that provides better protection against UV rays.

Use sunscreen: Apply a broad-spectrum sunscreen with a sun protection factor (SPF) of 30 or higher to all exposed skin, including your face, neck, and ears. Reapply every two hours or more frequently if you are swimming or sweating.

Avoid tanning beds: Tanning beds emit UV radiation that can increase the risk of skin cancer. Opt for sunless tanning products if you desire a tan.

6.3.5 Get Vaccinated

Certain viruses can increase the risk of developing cancer. Vaccines are available to protect against some of these viruses, including human papillomavirus (HPV) and hepatitis B. HPV is a sexually transmitted infection that can lead to cervical, anal, and other types of cancer. Hepatitis B is a viral infection that can cause liver cancer. By getting vaccinated, you can significantly reduce your risk of these types of cancer.

Talk to your healthcare provider about the recommended vaccines for your age group and individual risk factors. Vaccinations are a safe and effective way to prevent infections and reduce the risk of associated cancers.

6.3.6 Regular Screening and Early Detection

Regular cancer screenings can help detect cancer at an early stage when it is most treatable. Screening tests can vary depending on the type of cancer, age, and individual risk factors. Some common cancer screenings include mammograms for breast cancer, colonoscopies for colorectal cancer, and Pap tests for cervical cancer.

It is important to discuss with your healthcare provider about the appropriate screening tests for

your age and risk factors. By detecting cancer early, treatment options are often more effective, and the chances of survival are significantly improved.
Conclusion

Reducing the risk of cancer is a lifelong commitment to maintaining a healthy lifestyle. By adopting a healthy diet, maintaining a healthy weight, quitting smoking, protecting yourself from the sun, getting vaccinated, and undergoing regular screenings, you can significantly lower your risk of developing cancer as you age. Remember, prevention is key, and taking proactive steps today can lead to a healthier and longer life tomorrow.

6.4 MANAGING CHRONIC CONDITIONS

As we age, it is common for chronic conditions to develop. Chronic conditions are long-term health conditions that require ongoing management and care. These conditions can significantly impact our quality of life and overall well-being. However, with proper management and lifestyle modifications, it is possible to live well with chronic conditions and minimize their impact on our daily lives.

6.4.1 Understanding Chronic Conditions

Chronic conditions can encompass a wide range of health issues, including diabetes, arthritis, hypertension, heart disease, chronic obstructive pulmonary disease (COPD), and many others. These conditions often require ongoing medical treatment, medication, and lifestyle modifications to manage symptoms and prevent further complications.

It is important to understand the nature of your specific chronic condition and how it affects your body. Educating yourself about the condition can help you make informed decisions about your treatment plan and lifestyle modifications. Consult with your healthcare provider to gain a better understanding of your condition, its progression, and the best strategies for managing it.

6.4.2 Working with Healthcare Professionals

Managing chronic conditions requires a collaborative approach between you and your healthcare team. Your primary care physician, specialists, and other healthcare professionals play a crucial role in helping you manage your condition effectively.

Regular check-ups and appointments with your healthcare provider are essential for monitoring your condition, adjusting medications if necessary, and addressing any concerns or questions you may have. It is important to communicate openly and honestly with your healthcare team, sharing any changes in symptoms or concerns that may arise.

6.4.3 Medication Management

For many chronic conditions, medication is a key component of the treatment plan. It is important to take your medications as prescribed by your healthcare provider and to follow any specific instructions regarding dosage and timing. Adhering to your medication regimen can help control symptoms, prevent complications, and improve your overall health.

It is also important to be aware of potential side effects and interactions with other medications or supplements you may be taking. Always consult with your healthcare provider before starting any new medications or supplements to ensure they are safe and compatible with your current treatment plan.

6.4.4 Lifestyle Modifications

In addition to medication management, lifestyle modifications can play a significant role in managing chronic conditions. Making healthy choices in areas such as diet, exercise, stress management, and sleep can help improve symptoms, reduce the risk of complications, and enhance overall well-being.

Diet: A balanced and nutritious diet is essential for managing chronic conditions. Focus on consuming a variety of fruits, vegetables, whole grains, lean proteins, and healthy fats. Limit the intake of processed foods, sugary beverages, and foods high in saturated fats and sodium. Consult with a registered dietitian or nutritionist to develop a personalized meal plan that meets your specific dietary needs.

Exercise: Regular physical activity can help manage symptoms, improve cardiovascular health, and enhance overall well-being. Engage in activities that you enjoy and that are appropriate for your condition. Consult with your healthcare provider or a certified exercise specialist to develop an exercise routine that is safe and effective for you.

Stress Management: Chronic conditions can be stressful, and stress can exacerbate symptoms. Incorporate stress management techniques such as deep breathing exercises, meditation, yoga, or engaging in hobbies and activities that bring you joy and relaxation. Consider seeking support from a therapist or counselor who specializes in chronic illness management.

Sleep: Quality sleep is crucial for overall health and well-being. Establish a regular sleep routine, create a comfortable sleep environment, and practice good sleep hygiene habits. If you are experiencing sleep disturbances related to your chronic condition, consult with your healthcare provider for guidance and potential solutions.

6.4.5 Support Systems and Self-Care

Living with a chronic condition can be challenging, both physically and emotionally. It is important to build a strong support system and prioritize self-care to maintain a positive outlook and cope with the daily demands of managing your condition.

Seek support from family, friends, or support groups who understand and can empathize with your experiences. Sharing your journey with others who are going through similar challenges can provide a sense of community and validation.

Engage in activities that bring you joy and fulfillment. Take time for self-care, whether it's practicing mindfulness, engaging in hobbies, or pursuing creative outlets. Prioritizing self-care can help reduce stress, improve mental well-being, and enhance overall quality of life.

6.4.6 Regular Monitoring and Check-ups

Regular monitoring and check-ups are essential for managing chronic conditions effectively. Stay proactive in your healthcare by scheduling regular appointments with your healthcare provider, even if you are feeling well. These appointments allow for ongoing assessment of your condition, adjustment of treatment plans if necessary, and early detection of any potential complications.

Additionally, monitoring your symptoms and keeping track of any changes or patterns can provide valuable information for your healthcare team. Consider keeping a journal or using digital tools to track symptoms, medication adherence, and lifestyle factors that may impact your condition.

6.4.7 Embracing a Positive Mindset

Managing chronic conditions can be challenging, but maintaining a positive mindset can make a significant difference in your overall well-being. Embrace a mindset of resilience, focusing on what you can control and finding gratitude in the present moment. Surround yourself with positive influences and engage in activities that bring you joy and fulfillment.

Remember that managing chronic conditions is a journey, and it may require adjustments along the way. Stay open to new strategies, treatments, and technologies that may emerge in the future. With a proactive approach and a commitment to self-care, it is possible to live well with chronic conditions and continue aging with grace and purpose.

Managing chronic conditions is an integral part of aging well. By understanding your condition, working closely with your healthcare team, making lifestyle modifications, and prioritizing self-care, you can effectively manage your chronic condition and enhance your overall well-being. Remember to stay proactive, seek support, and maintain a positive mindset as you navigate the challenges and joys of aging with a chronic condition.

7. MAINTAINING A HEALTHY LIFESTYLE

7.1 MANAGING WEIGHT AND BODY COMPOSITION

Maintaining a healthy weight and body composition is crucial for aging well and promoting longevity. As we age, our metabolism slows down, and it becomes easier to gain weight and lose muscle mass. However, with the right strategies and lifestyle choices, it is possible to manage weight and body composition effectively.

7.1.1 Understanding the Importance of Weight Management

Managing weight is not just about appearance; it

is about overall health and well-being. Excess weight can increase the risk of various health conditions, including heart disease, diabetes, and certain types of cancer. Additionally, carrying extra weight can put strain on the joints and lead to mobility issues.

Maintaining a healthy weight can also improve energy levels, enhance cognitive function, and boost self-esteem. It is important to approach weight management with a focus on overall health rather than solely on achieving a specific number on the scale.

7.1.2 The Role of Nutrition in Weight Management

Nutrition plays a crucial role in managing weight and body composition. A balanced and nutrient-rich diet can help control appetite, provide essential nutrients, and support overall health. Here are some key principles to consider:

7.1.2.1 Caloric Balance

To manage weight effectively, it is important to maintain a caloric balance. This means consuming the right amount of calories to support your body's needs without exceeding them. Consuming more calories than your body requires can lead to weight gain, while consuming fewer calories can result in weight loss. It is essential to find the right balance that suits your individual needs and goals.

7.1.2.2 Macronutrient Distribution

The distribution of macronutrients, including carbohydrates, proteins, and fats, is important for weight management. A balanced diet should include a variety of nutrient-dense foods from all food groups. Carbohydrates provide energy, proteins support muscle growth and repair, and healthy fats are essential for various bodily functions. Finding the right balance of macronutrients can help control hunger, maintain muscle mass, and support overall health.

7.1.2.3 Portion Control

Portion control is another important aspect of weight management. It is easy to overeat when portion sizes are large or when we eat mindlessly. Being mindful of portion sizes and listening to your body's hunger and fullness cues can help prevent overeating and promote weight maintenance. Using smaller plates, measuring food portions, and being aware of serving sizes can all contribute to better portion control.

7.1.2.4 Nutrient Density

Choosing nutrient-dense foods is essential for managing weight and promoting overall health. Nutrient-dense foods are rich in vitamins, minerals, and other beneficial compounds while being relatively low in calories. Filling your plate with fruits, vegetables, whole grains, lean proteins, and healthy fats can help you feel satisfied while providing essential nutrients.

7.1.3 The Role of Physical Activity in Weight Management

In addition to nutrition, physical activity plays a vital role in managing weight and body composition. Regular exercise helps burn calories, build muscle mass, and improve overall fitness. Here are some key points to consider:

7.1.3.1 Aerobic Exercise

Engaging in aerobic exercises such as walking, jogging, swimming, or cycling can help burn calories and promote weight loss. Aim for at least 150 minutes of moderate-intensity aerobic activity or 75 minutes of vigorous-intensity aerobic activity per week. Incorporating activities that you enjoy and can sustain in the long term is important for adherence and overall success.

7.1.3.2 Strength Training

Including strength training exercises in your routine is crucial for maintaining and building muscle mass. As we age, we naturally lose muscle mass, which can lead to a decrease in metabolism. Strength training exercises, such as lifting weights or using resistance bands, can help preserve muscle mass, increase strength, and boost metabolism. Aim for two or more days of strength training per week, targeting all major muscle groups.

7.1.3.3 Physical Activity Throughout the Day

In addition to structured exercise sessions, it is important to incorporate physical activity throughout the day. Simple activities like taking the stairs instead of the elevator, walking or biking instead of driving, and engaging in household chores can all contribute to increased calorie expenditure and improved overall fitness.

7.1.4 Strategies for Successful Weight Management

Managing weight and body composition requires a holistic approach that combines nutrition, physical activity, and lifestyle choices. Here are some strategies to help you succeed:

7.1.4.1 Set Realistic Goals

Setting realistic and achievable goals is essential for long-term success. Instead of focusing on drastic weight loss, aim for gradual and sustainable changes. Set specific goals related to nutrition and physical activity, such as incorporating more vegetables into your meals or increasing your daily step count.

7.1.4.2 Practice Mindful Eating

Mindful eating involves paying attention to your body's hunger and fullness cues, as well as the sensory experience of eating. Slow down, savor each bite, and listen to your body's signals of hunger and satisfaction. Avoid distractions while eating, such as watching TV or using electronic devices, as this can lead to mindless overeating.

7.1.4.3 Seek Support

Having a support system can greatly enhance your weight management journey. Consider joining a support group, seeking guidance from a registered dietitian or a personal trainer, or involving friends and family in your healthy lifestyle changes. Support and accountability can help you stay motivated and overcome challenges.

7.1.4.4 Prioritize Sleep and Stress Management

Adequate sleep and effective stress management are crucial for weight management. Lack of sleep can disrupt hunger and satiety hormones, leading to increased appetite and cravings. Additionally, chronic stress can contribute to emotional eating and hinder weight loss efforts. Prioritize quality sleep and incorporate stress-reducing activities such as meditation, yoga, or hobbies into your routine.

Managing weight and body composition is an

important aspect of aging well and promoting longevity. By adopting a balanced and nutrient-rich diet, engaging in regular physical activity, and implementing healthy lifestyle habits, you can effectively manage your weight and support overall health as you age. Remember to approach weight management with a focus on overall well-being rather than solely on achieving a specific number on the scale.

7.2 MAINTAINING BONE HEALTH

As we age, it becomes increasingly important to prioritize the health of our bones. Maintaining strong and healthy bones is crucial for overall well-being and can help prevent conditions such as osteoporosis and fractures. In this section, we will explore the factors that contribute to bone health and discuss strategies for maintaining strong bones as we age.

7.2.1 Understanding Bone Health

Bones are living tissues that undergo a constant process of remodeling throughout our lives. This process involves the breakdown of old bone tissue and the formation of new bone tissue. However, as we age, this balance can be disrupted, leading to a loss of bone density and strength.

One of the key factors that affect bone health is the level of calcium and other minerals in our bodies. Calcium is essential for the formation and maintenance of strong bones. It is important to ensure an adequate intake of calcium through our diet or supplements, especially as we age. Other minerals, such as magnesium and phosphorus, also play a role in maintaining bone health.

Hormones, particularly estrogen and testosterone, also have a significant impact on bone health. Estrogen helps protect bone density in women, and the decline in estrogen levels during menopause can lead to a rapid loss of bone mass. Similarly, testosterone plays a role in maintaining bone density in men, and a decline in testosterone levels can contribute to bone loss.

7.2.2 Strategies for Maintaining Bone Health

Adequate Calcium Intake: Consuming enough calcium is essential for maintaining bone health. Good dietary sources of calcium include dairy products, leafy green vegetables, and fortified foods. If it is challenging to meet the recommended daily intake through diet alone, calcium supplements may be considered. It is important to consult with a healthcare professional before starting any new supplements.

Vitamin D: Vitamin D is crucial for the absorption of calcium in the body. Spending time outdoors and getting sunlight exposure can help the body produce vitamin D naturally. Additionally, certain foods such as fatty fish, fortified dairy products, and egg yolks are good dietary sources of vitamin D. In some cases, vitamin D supplements may be recommended, especially for individuals with limited sun exposure or specific medical conditions.

Regular Weight-Bearing Exercise: Engaging in weight-bearing exercises, such as walking, jogging, dancing, or weightlifting, can help stimulate bone growth and maintain bone density. These activities put stress on the bones, which signals the body to build stronger bones. It is important to choose exercises that are appropriate for your fitness level and consult with a healthcare professional before starting a new exercise program.

Avoid Smoking and Limit Alcohol Consumption: Smoking and excessive alcohol consumption can have detrimental effects on bone health. Smoking has been linked to a higher risk of fractures and lower bone density. Excessive alcohol consumption can interfere with the body's ability to absorb calcium and other essential nutrients for bone health. It is advisable to quit smoking and limit alcohol intake to promote optimal bone health.

Maintain a Healthy Body Weight: Maintaining a

healthy body weight is important for overall health, including bone health. Being underweight can increase the risk of bone loss and fractures, while being overweight can put excess stress on the bones. Striving for a balanced diet and regular exercise can help achieve and maintain a healthy weight.

Regular Bone Density Testing: Regular bone density testing, such as a dual-energy X-ray absorptiometry (DXA) scan, can help assess bone health and detect any signs of osteoporosis or bone loss. This can help identify potential issues early on and allow for appropriate interventions.

Consider Hormone Replacement Therapy: For individuals experiencing significant bone loss due to hormonal changes, hormone replacement therapy (HRT) may be considered. HRT involves the use of medications to supplement declining hormone levels and can help maintain bone density. However, it is important to discuss the potential risks and benefits of HRT with a healthcare professional.

Ensure a Balanced Diet: A balanced diet that includes a variety of nutrients is essential for overall health, including bone health. In addition to calcium and vitamin D, it is important to consume adequate amounts of other essential nutrients such as magnesium, phosphorus, vitamin K, and vitamin C. These nutrients can be found in a wide range of foods, including fruits, vegetables, whole grains, lean proteins, and nuts.

By implementing these strategies, individuals can take proactive steps to maintain and improve their bone health as they age. It is important to remember that bone health is a lifelong process and requires ongoing attention and care. Consulting with a healthcare professional can provide personalized guidance and recommendations based on individual needs and circumstances.

7.3 OPTIMIZING HORMONAL BALANCE

Hormones play a crucial role in our overall health and well-being, and as we age, hormonal imbalances can have a significant impact on our quality of life. Hormones are chemical messengers that regulate various bodily functions, including metabolism, mood, sleep, and sexual function. As we get older, our hormone levels naturally decline, leading to a range of symptoms and health issues. However, by optimizing hormonal balance, we can mitigate these effects and promote healthy aging.

7.3.1 Understanding Hormonal Changes with Age

As we age, our bodies undergo various hormonal changes. For both men and women, the most well-known hormonal change is the decline in reproductive hormones, such as estrogen and testosterone. In women, this decline occurs during menopause, while in men, it is known as andropause. However, hormonal changes go beyond reproductive hormones and can affect other systems in the body.

For women, the decline in estrogen during menopause can lead to symptoms such as hot flashes, night sweats, mood swings, and vaginal dryness. In men, the decline in testosterone can result in fatigue, reduced libido, muscle loss, and mood changes. Additionally, both men and women may experience changes in thyroid hormone levels, which can affect metabolism and energy levels.

7.3.2 The Importance of Hormonal Balance

Maintaining hormonal balance is essential for overall health and well-being. Hormones act as messengers, communicating with different organs and tissues to regulate various bodily functions. When hormones are imbalanced, it can lead to a range of symptoms and health issues.

For example, imbalances in thyroid hormones can result in weight gain or difficulty losing weight, fatigue, and mood changes. Imbalances in reproductive hormones can cause fertility issues, sexual dysfunction, and mood disturbances. Hormonal imbalances can also contribute to the development of chronic conditions such as diabetes, cardiovascular disease, and osteoporosis.

7.3.3 Strategies for Optimizing Hormonal Balance

While hormonal changes are a natural part of the aging process, there are strategies we can implement to optimize hormonal balance and promote healthy aging. Here are some key strategies to consider:

7.3.3.1 Healthy Diet

A nutritious diet plays a crucial role in maintaining hormonal balance. Include a variety of whole foods such as fruits, vegetables, whole grains, lean proteins, and healthy fats in your diet. Avoid processed foods, sugary snacks, and excessive alcohol consumption, as they can disrupt hormonal balance. Additionally, certain foods, such as cruciferous vegetables (broccoli, cauliflower, kale), can support estrogen metabolism and balance.

7.3.3.2 Regular Exercise

Regular physical activity is not only beneficial for overall health but also for hormonal balance. Engaging in aerobic exercise, strength training, and flexibility exercises can help regulate hormone levels. Exercise can also improve insulin sensitivity, which is important for managing blood sugar levels and preventing diabetes. Aim for at least 150 minutes of moderate-intensity exercise or 75 minutes of vigorous-intensity exercise per week.

7.3.3.3 Stress Management

Chronic stress can disrupt hormonal balance and contribute to various health issues. Implement stress management techniques such as meditation, deep breathing exercises, yoga, or engaging in hobbies and activities that bring you joy. Prioritize self-care and make time for relaxation and rejuvenation.

7.3.3.4 Quality Sleep

Adequate sleep is crucial for hormonal balance. Aim for 7-9 hours of quality sleep each night. Create a sleep-friendly environment by keeping your bedroom cool, dark, and quiet. Establish a regular sleep routine and avoid electronic devices before bedtime, as they can interfere with sleep quality.

7.3.3.5 Hormone Replacement Therapy

In some cases, hormone replacement therapy (HRT) may be recommended to optimize hormonal balance. HRT involves replacing deficient hormones with synthetic or bioidentical hormones to alleviate symptoms and improve overall well-being. However, HRT should be discussed with a healthcare professional, as it carries potential risks and benefits that need to be carefully considered.

7.3.4 Monitoring Hormonal Balance

Regular monitoring of hormone levels is important for optimizing hormonal balance. If you are experiencing symptoms of hormonal imbalance or are concerned about your hormone levels, consult with a healthcare professional. They can perform hormone tests and provide guidance on appropriate interventions, such as lifestyle modifications or hormone replacement therapy if necessary.

Optimizing hormonal balance is crucial for healthy aging. By implementing strategies such as maintaining a healthy diet, engaging in regular exercise, managing stress, prioritizing quality sleep, and considering hormone replacement therapy when appropriate, we can support our overall well-being and promote healthy aging. Regular monitoring of hormone levels and consulting with healthcare professionals can ensure that any imbalances are addressed promptly. Remember, hormonal balance is an essential component of the longevity blueprint for aging well.

7.4 HEALTHY AGING HABITS

As we age, it becomes increasingly important to adopt healthy habits that can support our overall well-being and promote longevity. In this section, we will explore some key habits that can contribute to healthy aging and provide practical tips for incorporating them into your daily routine.

7.4.1 Stay Physically Active

Regular physical activity is crucial for maintaining optimal health as we age. Engaging in exercise not only helps to keep our bodies strong and flexible but also has numerous benefits for our mental and emotional well-being. Aim for at least 150 minutes of moderate-intensity aerobic activity per week, such as brisk walking, swimming, or cycling. Additionally, incorporate strength training exercises at least twice a week to maintain muscle mass and bone density.

7.4.2 Eat a Balanced Diet

Nutrition plays a vital role in healthy aging. A well-balanced diet rich in fruits, vegetables, whole grains, lean proteins, and healthy fats can provide the necessary nutrients to support our body's functions and reduce the risk of chronic diseases. Include a variety of colorful fruits and vegetables in your meals, opt for whole grains instead of refined grains, choose lean sources of protein such as fish, poultry, and legumes, and incorporate healthy fats from sources like nuts, seeds, and olive oil.

7.4.3 Hydrate Properly

Staying hydrated is essential for maintaining optimal health, especially as we age. Dehydration can lead to various health issues, including fatigue, dizziness, and cognitive decline. Aim to drink at least eight glasses of water per day, and increase your fluid intake if you are physically active or in hot weather. Additionally, limit your consumption of sugary beverages and alcohol, as they can contribute to dehydration.

7.4.4 Get Sufficient Sleep

Adequate sleep is crucial for our overall health and well-being. As we age, our sleep patterns may change, and it may become more challenging to get a good night's sleep. However, prioritizing sleep is essential for healthy aging. Aim for seven to nine hours of quality sleep each night. Establish a relaxing bedtime routine, create a comfortable sleep environment, and limit the consumption of caffeine and electronic devices before bed to promote better sleep.

7.4.5 Manage Stress

Chronic stress can have detrimental effects on our physical and mental health. Learning effective stress management techniques is crucial for healthy aging. Engage in activities that help you relax and unwind, such as meditation, deep breathing exercises, yoga, or spending time in nature. Additionally, prioritize self-care activities that bring you joy and help you recharge. Surround yourself with a supportive network of friends and family who can provide emotional support during challenging times.

7.4.6 Maintain Social Connections

Maintaining strong social connections is vital for healthy aging. Engaging in social activities and nurturing relationships can have a positive impact on our mental and emotional well-being. Make an effort to stay connected with friends, family, and community groups. Join clubs or organizations that align with your interests, volunteer for causes you care about, or participate in group activities or classes. Building and maintaining social connections can provide a sense of belonging and purpose, reducing the risk of loneliness and isolation.

7.4.7 Practice Brain-Boosting Activities

Keeping our minds active and engaged is essential for maintaining cognitive function as we age. Engage in activities that challenge your brain, such as puzzles, reading, learning a new skill or language, or playing strategic games. Additionally, consider incorporating mindfulness practices, such as meditation or journaling, to promote mental clarity and emotional well-being.

7.4.8 Prioritize Preventive Healthcare

Regular check-ups and preventive healthcare measures are crucial for detecting and managing potential health issues before they become more serious. Schedule regular visits with your healthcare provider, undergo recommended screenings and vaccinations, and follow any prescribed treatments or medications. Additionally, be proactive in managing your health by adopting healthy habits and making informed lifestyle choices.

7.4.9 Maintain a Positive Outlook

Maintaining a positive outlook and embracing a mindset of gratitude can have a significant impact on our overall well-being as we age. Cultivate a positive attitude, focus on the present moment, and practice gratitude for the blessings in your life. Surround yourself with positive influences and engage in activities that bring you joy and fulfillment. Embracing a positive mindset can help reduce stress, enhance resilience, and promote a sense of purpose and fulfillment.

Incorporating these healthy aging habits into your daily routine can have a profound impact on your overall well-being and promote longevity.

Remember that it's never too late to start adopting these habits, and small changes can make a significant difference in your health and quality of life as you age. Embrace the journey of healthy aging and enjoy the benefits of a long and fulfilling life.

8. LONGEVITY STRATEGIES FOR THE FUTURE

8.1 ADVANCEMENTS IN ANTI-AGING RESEARCH

As our understanding of aging continues to evolve, so does the field of anti-aging research. Scientists and researchers are constantly exploring new avenues and technologies to slow down the aging process and extend human lifespan. In this chapter, we will delve into some of the exciting advancements in anti-aging research and the potential they hold for the future of longevity.

8.1.1 Telomeres and Telomerase

Telomeres, the protective caps at the ends of our chromosomes, play a crucial role in cellular aging. With each cell division, telomeres naturally shorten, eventually leading to cellular senescence and aging. However, recent research has focused on the enzyme telomerase, which has the ability to lengthen telomeres and potentially reverse the aging process.

Studies have shown that activating telomerase in laboratory animals can extend their lifespan and improve their overall health. While telomerase therapy is still in its early stages, it holds promise for future anti-aging interventions. Researchers are exploring various approaches to safely and effectively activate telomerase in humans, with the hope of slowing down the aging process and preventing age-related diseases.

8.1.2 Senescence and Senolytics

Cellular senescence, the state in which cells lose their ability to divide and function properly, is a hallmark of aging. Senescent cells accumulate in our bodies over time and contribute to age-related diseases and the overall decline in health. However, recent advancements in anti-aging research have focused on targeting and eliminating these senescent cells through a process called senolysis.

Senolytics are drugs or compounds that

selectively kill senescent cells, allowing healthier cells to thrive. This approach has shown promising results in animal studies, improving healthspan and delaying the onset of age-related diseases. Researchers are now working on developing senolytic therapies for human use, with the potential to revolutionize the field of anti-aging medicine.

8.1.3 Genetic Manipulation and Epigenetics

Advancements in genetic manipulation and epigenetics have opened up new possibilities for extending human lifespan. Scientists are exploring the role of specific genes and epigenetic modifications in the aging process, with the aim of developing interventions that can slow down or reverse aging.

One area of interest is the SIRT family of genes, which are involved in regulating cellular processes related to aging. Activation of these genes through caloric restriction or the use of certain compounds has been shown to extend lifespan in various organisms. Researchers are now investigating the potential of SIRT activators as anti-aging interventions in humans.

Epigenetic modifications, which can influence gene expression without altering the underlying DNA sequence, also play a crucial role in aging. Researchers are studying the impact of lifestyle factors, such as diet and exercise, on epigenetic changes and their effects on aging. Understanding these mechanisms could lead to personalized anti-aging strategies based on an individual's unique epigenetic profile.

8.1.4 Stem Cells and Regenerative Medicine

Stem cells have long been a topic of interest in anti-aging research. These unique cells have the ability to differentiate into various cell types and regenerate damaged tissues. As we age, the regenerative capacity of our stem cells declines, leading to impaired tissue repair and increased susceptibility to age-related diseases.

Scientists are exploring ways to harness the regenerative potential of stem cells to rejuvenate aging tissues and organs. Stem cell therapies, such as the transplantation of young stem cells or the activation of endogenous stem cells, hold promise for reversing the effects of aging and restoring youthful function. While still in the experimental stage, regenerative medicine approaches are a rapidly advancing field with the potential to revolutionize the way we age.

8.1.5 Artificial Intelligence and Machine Learning

Artificial intelligence (AI) and machine learning have become powerful tools in anti-aging research. These technologies can analyze vast amounts of data and identify patterns and correlations that may not be apparent to human researchers. AI algorithms can help predict the risk of age-related diseases, identify potential drug targets, and optimize personalized anti-aging interventions.

Researchers are also using AI to develop aging clocks, which are algorithms that can accurately estimate an individual's biological age based on various molecular markers. These clocks can provide valuable insights into the aging process and help monitor the effectiveness of anti-aging interventions.

8.1.6 Ethical Considerations and Future Implications

While the advancements in anti-aging research hold great promise, they also raise important ethical considerations. The pursuit of longevity should not come at the expense of quality of life or exacerbate existing social inequalities. It is crucial to ensure that these technologies and therapies are accessible, affordable, and used responsibly.

8.2 LONGEVITY TECHNOLOGIES AND THERAPIES

As we continue to explore the possibilities of extending human lifespan, advancements in technology and therapies are playing a crucial role. Longevity technologies and therapies are emerging as promising tools in the quest for healthy aging and increased lifespan. In this section, we will delve into some of the most exciting developments in this field and how they can potentially enhance our longevity.

8.2.1 Telomere Lengthening

Telomeres, the protective caps at the ends of our chromosomes, play a vital role in cellular aging. As we age, our telomeres naturally shorten, leading to cellular dysfunction and increased risk of age-related diseases. Telomere lengthening therapies aim to slow down or reverse this process, potentially extending our lifespan.

One approach to telomere lengthening is through the activation of telomerase, an enzyme that can rebuild and lengthen telomeres. Researchers are exploring various methods to stimulate telomerase activity, including the use of small molecules, gene therapy, and stem cell-based treatments. While these approaches are still in the experimental stage, they hold great promise for the future of longevity.

8.2.2 Senolytics

Senescence, the state of irreversible cell cycle arrest, is a hallmark of aging. Senescent cells accumulate in our bodies over time and contribute to age-related diseases and the overall decline in health. Senolytics are a class of drugs that target and eliminate these senescent cells, potentially rejuvenating tissues and organs.

Several senolytic compounds have shown promising results in preclinical and early clinical trials. These compounds selectively induce apoptosis (cell death) in senescent cells, clearing them from the body. By removing these harmful cells, senolytics have the potential to improve tissue function, delay age-related diseases, and enhance overall healthspan.

8.2.3 Genetic Interventions

Advancements in genetic engineering and gene editing technologies have opened up new possibilities for extending human lifespan. Scientists are exploring various genetic interventions that could potentially slow down the aging process and increase longevity.

One approach is the manipulation of specific genes involved in aging pathways. By targeting genes such as mTOR, AMPK, and SIRT1, researchers aim to mimic the effects of caloric restriction, a well-known method for extending lifespan in various organisms. These interventions could potentially enhance cellular repair mechanisms, improve metabolic health, and delay age-related decline.

Another area of genetic intervention is the use of CRISPR-Cas9 technology to edit the genome and correct age-related mutations. This revolutionary gene editing tool holds immense potential for treating genetic diseases and potentially slowing down the aging process. While still in its early stages, CRISPR-Cas9 has shown promising results in animal studies and offers hope for future therapeutic applications in humans.

8.2.4 Hormone Replacement Therapies

Hormones play a crucial role in regulating various physiological processes in our bodies. As we age, hormone levels decline, leading to a range of age-related symptoms and health issues. Hormone replacement therapies aim to restore hormone levels to a more youthful state, potentially improving overall health and longevity.

One well-known hormone replacement therapy is estrogen replacement for postmenopausal women. Estrogen therapy has been shown to alleviate menopausal symptoms, reduce the risk of osteoporosis, and potentially lower the risk of cardiovascular disease. However, hormone replacement therapies should be approached with caution and under the guidance of a healthcare professional, as they can have both benefits and risks.

8.2.5 Caloric Restriction Mimetics

Caloric restriction, the practice of reducing calorie intake without malnutrition, has been shown to extend lifespan and improve health in various organisms. However, practicing caloric restriction in humans can be challenging and may not be suitable for everyone. Caloric restriction mimetics are compounds that mimic the effects of caloric restriction without the need for drastic dietary changes.

Several caloric restriction mimetics, such as resveratrol and rapamycin, have shown promising results in animal studies. These compounds activate cellular pathways that promote longevity and improve metabolic health. While more research is needed to determine their efficacy and safety in humans, caloric restriction mimetics hold potential as a non-invasive approach to promoting healthy aging.

8.2.6 Personalized Medicine and Biomarkers

Advancements in personalized medicine and the identification of biomarkers are revolutionizing the field of longevity. Personalized medicine takes into account an individual's unique genetic makeup, lifestyle factors, and health history to tailor preventive and therapeutic interventions.

Biomarkers, measurable indicators of biological processes, provide valuable insights into an individual's health status and aging trajectory. By identifying specific biomarkers associated with aging and age-related diseases, researchers can develop targeted interventions to slow down the aging process and prevent age-related decline.

The integration of personalized medicine and biomarkers holds great promise for the future of longevity. By understanding an individual's unique genetic and biological makeup, healthcare professionals can develop personalized interventions that optimize health, prevent disease, and promote longevity.

In conclusion, longevity technologies and therapies are rapidly advancing, offering exciting possibilities for extending human lifespan and promoting healthy aging. From telomere lengthening to genetic interventions and personalized medicine, these advancements have the potential to revolutionize the way we approach aging. While many of these technologies are still in the experimental stage, they provide hope for a future where aging is not only understood but also actively managed to enhance our quality of life and increase our years of healthy living.

8.3 PLANNING FOR A LONG AND HEALTHY LIFE

As we age, it becomes increasingly important to plan for a long and healthy life. While we cannot control all aspects of the aging process, there are steps we can take to optimize our health and well-being as we grow older. In this section, we will explore some key strategies for planning and preparing for a fulfilling and vibrant future.

8.3.1 Setting Goals for Healthy Aging

One of the first steps in planning for a long and healthy life is to set clear goals. By identifying what we want to achieve and the areas of our health and well-being that are most important to us, we can create a roadmap for success. These goals may include maintaining physical fitness, preserving cognitive function, nurturing social connections, and preventing age-related diseases.

When setting goals, it is important to make them specific, measurable, achievable, relevant, and time-bound (SMART). For example, instead of setting a vague goal like "I want to be healthier," a SMART goal could be "I will engage in moderate-intensity aerobic exercise for 30 minutes, five days a week, to improve cardiovascular health and maintain a healthy weight."

8.3.2 Creating a Long-Term Health Plan

Once we have established our goals, it is essential to create a long-term health plan. This plan should encompass various aspects of our well-being, including nutrition, exercise, mental health, sleep, and preventive care. By addressing these areas comprehensively, we can maximize our chances of aging well and enjoying a high quality of life.

When developing a long-term health plan, it is helpful to consult with healthcare professionals, such as doctors, nutritionists, and fitness trainers. They can provide valuable guidance and tailor the plan to our specific needs and circumstances. Additionally, it is important to regularly review and update the plan as our health needs and goals may change over time.

8.3.3 Prioritizing Preventive Care

Preventive care plays a crucial role in planning for a long and healthy life. Regular check-ups, screenings, and vaccinations can help detect and prevent potential health issues before they become more serious. It is important to follow recommended guidelines for preventive care, such as getting regular physical exams, mammograms, colonoscopies, and vaccinations.

In addition to medical preventive care, it is also important to prioritize lifestyle factors that can reduce the risk of age-related diseases. This includes maintaining a healthy diet, engaging in regular exercise, managing stress, getting enough sleep, and avoiding harmful habits such as smoking and excessive alcohol consumption.

8.3.4 Financial Planning for Longevity

Planning for a long and healthy life also involves considering the financial aspects of aging. As we age, healthcare costs and other expenses may increase. It is important to assess our financial situation and develop a plan to ensure we have the resources to support our health and well-being in the future.

This may involve saving for retirement, exploring long-term care insurance options, and considering estate planning. Consulting with a financial advisor can provide valuable insights and help us make informed decisions about our financial future.

8.3.5 Cultivating a Positive Mindset

In addition to physical and financial planning, cultivating a positive mindset is essential for aging well. Embracing the aging process with grace and purpose can significantly impact our overall well-being. It is important to let go of societal expectations and embrace the wisdom and experience that come with age.

Practicing gratitude, mindfulness, and self-compassion can help us navigate the challenges and changes that come with aging. Surrounding ourselves with a supportive community and engaging in meaningful activities can also contribute to a positive mindset and a sense of purpose.

8.3.6 Adapting to Change

As we age, it is important to be flexible and adaptable to the changes that may occur. Our health needs and abilities may evolve, and it is crucial to adjust our plans and expectations accordingly. This may involve modifying our exercise routine, seeking new social connections, or exploring new hobbies and interests.

By embracing change and being open to new possibilities, we can continue to grow and thrive as we age. It is important to approach each stage of life with curiosity and a willingness to learn and adapt.

8.3.7 Building a Supportive Network

Building a supportive network is vital for planning a long and healthy life. Surrounding ourselves with positive and like-minded individuals can provide emotional support, motivation, and a sense of belonging. This network can include family, friends, healthcare professionals, and community groups.

Maintaining strong social connections can help combat feelings of loneliness and isolation, which are common among older adults. Regularly engaging in social activities, volunteering, and participating in group activities can foster meaningful connections and contribute to overall well-being.

8.3.8 Continual Learning and Personal Growth

Finally, planning for a long and healthy life involves a commitment to continual learning and personal growth. Engaging in intellectual pursuits, learning new skills, and staying curious can help keep our minds sharp and our spirits young. This can include reading books, taking courses, attending lectures, or exploring new hobbies.

By embracing lifelong learning, we can continue to expand our horizons, challenge ourselves, and find fulfillment in the pursuit of knowledge and personal growth.

Planning for a long and healthy life involves

setting goals, creating a comprehensive health plan, prioritizing preventive care, considering financial aspects, cultivating a positive mindset, adapting to change, building a supportive network, and committing to continual learning and personal growth. By taking proactive steps and embracing the aging process with intention and purpose, we can increase our chances of aging well and enjoying a fulfilling and vibrant future.

8.4 EMBRACING AGING WITH GRACE AND PURPOSE

As we journey through life, it is inevitable that we will age. However, aging does not have to be something to fear or dread. In fact, it can be a time of great fulfillment, wisdom, and joy. Embracing aging with grace and purpose is about accepting the natural process of getting older while finding meaning and fulfillment in every stage of life. In this final chapter, we will explore the mindset and attitudes that can help us embrace aging with grace and purpose.

8.4.1 Cultivating a Positive Mindset

One of the most important aspects of embracing aging with grace and purpose is cultivating a positive mindset. Our thoughts and beliefs have a powerful impact on our overall well-being.

Research has shown that individuals with a positive outlook on aging tend to live longer, healthier lives. So how can we cultivate a positive mindset as we age?

Firstly, it is important to challenge negative stereotypes and societal expectations about aging. Many people hold onto outdated beliefs that aging is synonymous with decline and loss. However, research has shown that older adults can continue to learn, grow, and contribute to society in meaningful ways. By challenging these negative stereotypes, we can create a more positive and empowering narrative around aging.

Secondly, practicing gratitude can greatly enhance our overall well-being as we age. Taking time each day to reflect on the things we are grateful for can shift our focus from what we may have lost to what we still have. Gratitude helps us appreciate the present moment and find joy in the simple pleasures of life.

8.4.2 Finding Purpose and Meaning

Another key aspect of embracing aging with grace and purpose is finding meaning and purpose in our lives. As we age, it is common to experience a shift in priorities and goals. This can be an opportunity to reflect on what truly matters to us and how we can make a positive impact on the world around us.

Finding purpose and meaning can take many forms. It may involve pursuing a new hobby or passion, volunteering for a cause we care about, or mentoring younger generations. Engaging in activities that align with our values and bring us joy can give us a sense of purpose and fulfillment.

Additionally, maintaining social connections and nurturing relationships is crucial for finding meaning in our lives as we age. Building and maintaining strong relationships with family, friends, and community members can provide a sense of belonging and support. Engaging in meaningful conversations, sharing experiences, and offering support to others can bring a deep sense of purpose and fulfillment.

8.4.3 Self-Care and Well-being

Taking care of ourselves physically, mentally, and emotionally is essential for embracing aging with grace and purpose. Self-care practices can help us maintain our overall well-being and enhance our quality of life as we age.

Physical self-care involves engaging in regular exercise, eating a balanced diet, and getting enough restful sleep. Staying active can help maintain strength, flexibility, and mobility, while a nutritious diet provides the necessary nutrients for optimal health. Prioritizing sleep is also important, as it allows our bodies and minds to rejuvenate and repair.

Mental and emotional self-care involves managing stress, practicing mindfulness, and seeking support when needed. Chronic stress can have detrimental effects on our health, so finding healthy coping mechanisms such as meditation, deep breathing exercises, or engaging in activities we enjoy can help reduce stress levels. Seeking support from loved ones or professional counselors can also provide valuable guidance and assistance during challenging times.

8.4.4 Embracing Change and Adaptability

As we age, it is important to embrace change and cultivate adaptability. Life is full of transitions, and being open to new experiences and perspectives can greatly enhance our well-being. Embracing change involves letting go of rigid expectations and embracing the opportunities that come with each new phase of life.

Adaptability is also crucial for navigating the challenges that may arise as we age. It involves being open to learning new skills, adjusting to physical and cognitive changes, and finding creative solutions to overcome obstacles. By embracing change and cultivating adaptability, we can approach aging with a sense of curiosity and resilience.

8.4.5 Embracing Aging as a Journey

Finally, embracing aging with grace and purpose is about viewing it as a journey rather than a destination. Each stage of life brings its own unique joys, challenges, and opportunities for growth. By embracing the present moment and finding meaning in every experience, we can fully appreciate the richness and depth of the aging process.

Remember, aging is a natural part of life, and it is up to us to make the most of it. By cultivating a positive mindset, finding purpose and meaning, practicing self-care, embracing change and adaptability, and viewing aging as a journey, we can embrace the process of getting older with grace and purpose. Let us embark on this journey with open hearts and minds, ready to embrace all that life has to offer.

CONCLUSION

In concluding our exploration of aging well in "Aging Well: The Longevity Blueprint," we arrive at a juncture where knowledge meets action, and wisdom converges with daily choices. The journey through these pages has been a venture into the intricacies of longevity, guided by the latest scientific insights and a commitment to straightforward, actionable advice.

As we reflect on the comprehensive blueprint laid out before you, it becomes clear that aging is not a singular destination but a dynamic process, continually shaped by the choices we make. The culmination of our exploration reveals a tapestry woven with the threads of nutrition, exercise, mental health, sleep, and disease prevention—a tapestry that, when embraced intentionally, has the power to enrich and extend the chapters of our lives.

Our discussion on nutrition illuminated the profound impact of what we consume on our overall well-being. From essential nutrients to mindful meal planning, the choices we make at the table play a pivotal role in supporting our bodies as they age.

The role of exercise emerged as a cornerstone in the pursuit of longevity, showcasing the transformative power of movement on both our physical and mental health. Whether through structured routines or everyday activities, the benefits of staying active reverberate throughout the years.

Mental health, often overlooked in discussions on aging, took center stage, emphasizing the importance of cognitive function, stress management, and nurturing emotional well-being. The acknowledgement of social connections as a vital aspect of mental health further underscored the interconnected nature of our well-being.

The significance of sleep in our quest for a fulfilling life cannot be overstated. Our exploration of sleep uncovered practical solutions for improving sleep quality, allowing for rejuvenation and vitality to permeate our waking hours.

Disease prevention and the management of chronic conditions emerged as critical components of aging well. By understanding and addressing these challenges, we empower ourselves to take charge of our health and preserve the quality of our lives.

Advancements in anti-aging research and longevity technologies provided a glimpse into the exciting possibilities that lie on the horizon, inviting us to consider not just the present but the potential of a future marked by vitality and innovation.

As we bid farewell to these pages, we do so with the conviction that aging is not a foe to be battled but a journey to be navigated with intention and purpose. Each passing year is an opportunity to celebrate the wisdom gained, the resilience cultivated, and the beauty inherent in the passage of time.

May the knowledge within this blueprint serve as a compass as you chart your course through the years ahead. With every choice you make, may you continue to age well—embracing the fullness of life with grace, vitality, and the wisdom that only time can bestow.

This is not just the conclusion of a book; it is an invitation to embark on a lifelong journey of aging well, one choice at a time.